Sana Zakaryaie Nasab
Heman Dehghani
Shaghayegh Jamshidi Rastabi

Cancer and Lifestyle

Sana Zakaryaie Nasab
Heman Dehghani
Shaghayegh Jamshidi Rastabi

Cancer and Lifestyle

Noor Publishing

Imprint

Any brand names and product names mentioned in this book are subject to trademark, brand or patent protection and are trademarks or registered trademarks of their respective holders. The use of brand names, product names, common names, trade names, product descriptions etc. even without a particular marking in this work is in no way to be construed to mean that such names may be regarded as unrestricted in respect of trademark and brand protection legislation and could thus be used by anyone.

Cover image: www.ingimage.com

Publisher:
Noor Publishing
is a trademark of
Dodo Books Indian Ocean Ltd., member of the OmniScriptum S.R.L Publishing group
str. A.Russo 15, of. 61, Chisinau-2068, Republic of Moldova Europe
Printed at: see last page
ISBN: 978-620-3-86048-1

Cancer and Lifestyle

By

Sana Zakaryaie Nasab

Master of Internal Surgery Nursing Kurdestan University of Medical Sciences, Iran

Heman Dehghani

Master of Internal Surgery Nursing Kurdestan University of Medical Sciences, Iran

Shaghayegh Jamshidi Rastabi

Bachelor of Nursing, Master of Science in Medical-Surgical Nursing Shahrekord University of Medical science, Shahrekord, Iran

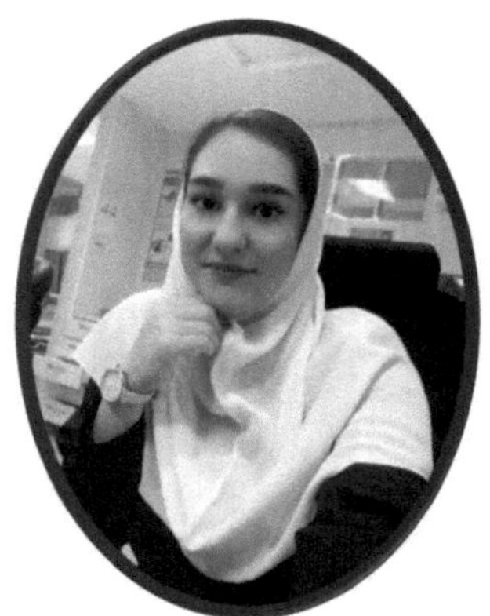

Sana Zakaryaie Nasab

Master of Internal Surgery Nursing Kurdestan University of
Medical Sciences, Iran

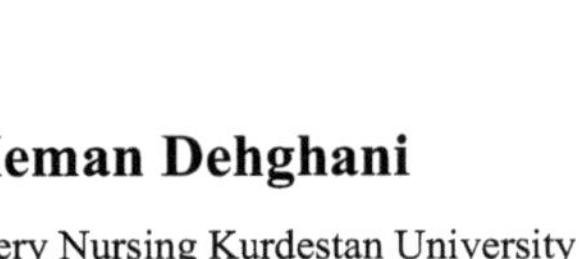

Heman Dehghani

Master of Internal Surgery Nursing Kurdestan University of Medical
Sciences, Iran

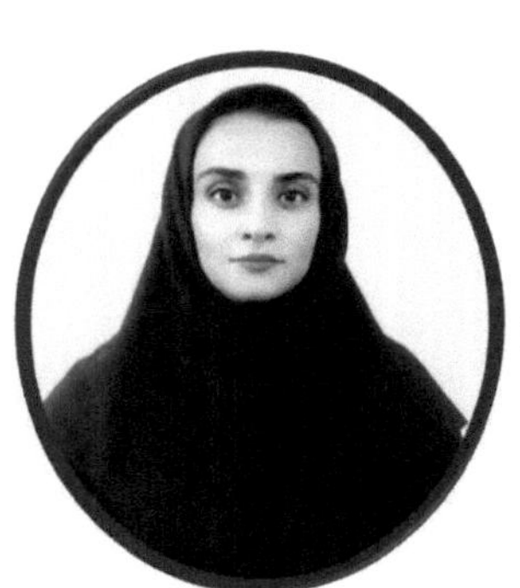

Shaghayegh Jamshidi Rastabi

Bachelor of Nursing, Master of Science In Medical-Surgical Nursing
Shahrekord University of Medical science, Shahrekord, Iran

This Book is dedicated to

My Family's

Content

Chapter I

Introduction

Introduction

Cancer as a bitter reality and an important stressor is a complication that changes the course of a person's life and increases the vulnerability and loss of quality of life, daily functions, social activities and the ability to perform roles. Changes the usual. In today's world, one of the most common causes of morbidity and mortality is due to cancer. According to the World Health Organization, the number of cancer deaths in the world will increase by 45% from 2007 to 2030 (from 7.9 million to 11.5 million deaths). More than half of all cancers occur in developing countries. Also, in most developing countries, cancer is the second leading cause of death after cardiovascular disease.

In Iran, as a developing country, cancer is the third leading cause of death after heart disease and road accidents. According to the results of Mousavi's study in 2006, the annual incidence of cancer among Iranian men and women is 98 and 110 per 100,000, respectively. Although cancer medically occurs in one person, family members contribute to the psychological and social problems of the disease. A diagnosis of cancer causes a major change in family life that Rolland refers to as an "uninvited guest" that must be accepted by the family or couple. At every stage of the disease, the family faces challenges that threaten lasting relationships and their quality of life.

It is widely accepted that the fight against cancer is a family affair. Not only the patient, but also everyone who loves him or her faces the consequences of illness and treatment, which may include disruption of daily life, anxiety, worries about cancer recurrence, fear of loss and death. When a family is confronted with a stressor, the family first mobilizes its resources to solve the problem. When trying to solve a problem fails, the family goes into crisis. When family resources are insufficient or depleted, family functioning deteriorates and symptoms of family turmoil, such as parental problems and conflict between individuals, occur.

Also, when the family does not receive any help from outside the system, the result appears in the form of lower levels of family functioning or perhaps separation and the loss of a member. The experience of a stressful life makes people vulnerable. Vulnerable families, such as families with a sick member, are more likely to develop health problems as a result of exposure to risk or worse consequences as a result of health problems.

As mentioned, families with a member with a severe illness that puts the family under stress are considered vulnerable families and, therefore, are considered as a target group for community health nurses. One of the main approaches to working with vulnerable families in community health nursing is the family approach as a client. In this approach, the primary focus is on the family and the secondary on individuals. In this approach, the focus is on how the family as a whole reacts when family members experience a health problem. In the family unit, any defective function (illness, separation, etc.) that affects one member affects the other members in various ways, as well as the family unit as a whole, which is often a "wave effect". It is also called. There is also a strong relationship between the family and its health status. Hence, the role of the family is very crucial in any form of care, from health promotion to rehabilitation.

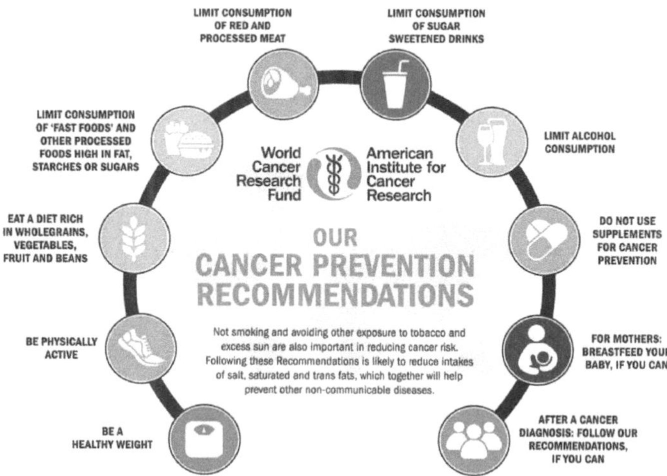

Figure 1. WCRF Provides Ten Lifestyle Recommendations to Reduce Cancer Risk

Family function means the ability of the family to adapt to changes made during life, conflict resolution, solidarity between members, implementation of the rules governing this institution, with the aim of maintaining the entire family system. Family performance shows how well the family works as a unit and also measures the family's ability to adapt and judge in different situations. It is necessary to evaluate families to have a theoretical model of how they function. One of the most useful models for examining the family is the McMaster model of family functioning and was developed in 1960 by Eptein and Lawrence. Although this model does not cover all aspects of family functioning, it does address important aspects that are often clinically evident. This model considers six aspects of family functioning: 1- Problem solving 2- Communication 3- Roles 4- Emotional responsiveness 5- Emotional mixing 6- Behavior control.

The McMaster model deals with the current functioning of the family, not with the evolutionary stage of the family or its previous growth. This model divides family responsibilities into three parts. Basic tasks such as providing food, security, health care for its members. Transformational tasks such as caring for the baby and caring for the adolescent in the family, critical tasks that include family skills in times of crisis and unexpected events such as the severe illness of a family member.

The important point is, why is it so important to work with the families of cancer patients? Northouse (2010), in a meta-analysis study of families of cancer patients in the United States, listed four reasons why families in cancer patients need to work: 1. When a member has cancer, members Her family is under considerable stress. 2. Family members often do not talk to each other about their thoughts and feelings about cancer. 3. Families try to cope with the effects of cancer and stress in the family, which is mainly due to cancer. They are created to adapt. 4. Family members try to maintain their original function.

The family is considered as the first source of support and care for a member with the disease and the attitude of the family towards cancer and its complications has a great impact on patient care. Depending on the role of the affected person in the family structure, the impact of cancer on family functioning will be different. The most important role to be considered in dealing with the family is the role of the parent. Diagnosis of cancer in parents' changes parental behavior, physical and mental functioning, as well as family functioning.

When parents are sick, the quality of medical care includes attention to the patient's role as a parent and the needs of their children. Maternal cancer can act as a stressor for the child.

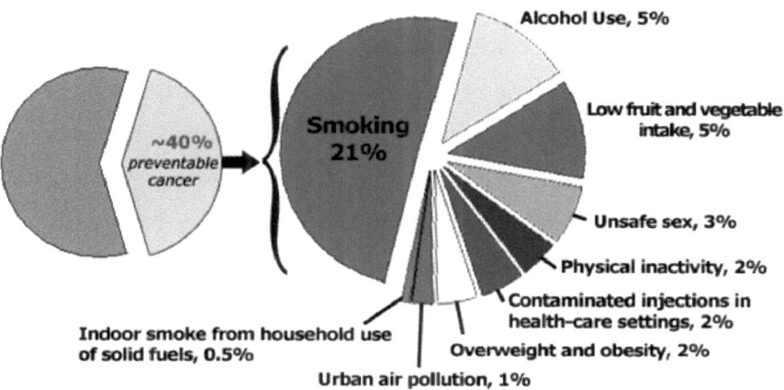

Figure 2. Cancer and Lifestyle

The results of the Schmitt study showed that there is dysfunction of families with parents with cancer, the most important cause being parental depression in the field of cancer, which in turn will have a negative impact on children's mental health, especially if another risk factor such as income There is little in the family. Sick parents are less able to care for family members, and as a result, children are forced to take on new tasks and roles, and such children may experience personality fluctuations in adulthood. Also, in Montaseri (2008) research on children with parents with cancer, the results have shown that the incidence of chronic diseases such as cancer in parents is associated with complications in family members, especially children. The impact of parental cancer diagnosis on children varies, not only because of differences in the age of the children, but also because of the type of cancer and the parents' hopes for long-term survival after cancer. Also, the complexities of treatment can affect the quality of life of children of parents with cancer. The results of a study conducted in the United States on the relationship between a couple during cancer in one of them have shown that when a couple gets cancer, their spouse is as stressed as he or she is. When men in the family get sick, their husbands are more stressed than when they are sick, because women often tend to carry the burden of care alone or without the help of others.

In addition, they must continue to do their daily chores and care for the children. The amount of stress that couples receive also depends on the stage of the disease. Couples, especially husbands, have the highest levels of stress in the final phase of the disease due to fear of recurrence. Experience cancer. Considering the duties of women and their social roles within the family, it has been found that women are more effective and active than men in maintaining the family unit. On the other hand, fathers of families have more disorders in roles and communication than mothers. Reproductive health problems, including impaired sexual function and impaired fertility, are also stressful and persist even after cancer treatment.

Processes within families proceed properly when members are able to play their expected roles. Roles go back to established patterns of behavior. One of the most important roles of a community health nurse in dealing with families in crisis is to help the family to use the abilities and resources of the family to fight the crisis. The family's ability to fight the crisis depends on family resources, including social resources (spouse, children, parents, siblings, etc.).

Cultural resources, religious resources, educational resources and medical resources. In Iran, despite the importance of the family in caring for cancer patients, scattered studies have been conducted on various aspects of the family and family functioning has been indirectly mentioned. One of these studies is the Photokian study in 2004, which examined only the quality of life of first-degree relatives of patients with cancer. Disorder and social isolation, financial problems, disruption of personal relationships and sexual relations with the spouse are observed.

Also, a 2008 study by Montaseri that identified the physical, psychological, and social problems of children with parents with cancer found that life-threatening illnesses in parents disrupted the normal family process and caused stress in members. It affects children in particular. No study in Iran has directly and comprehensively targeted the performance of families of cancer patients. But the most important variable that affects the health of any society is the social, economic, environmental, geographical, political and social status of that society.

Understanding the economic environment that affects the family is very important when trying to support the family system. To the extent that income is primarily important in terms of impact on family performance. Also, the amount of support available to families from government and non-government agencies in times of crisis varies in different communities. Ethnicity also affects how families respond to stressful situations and support each other. The results of Heydari's study also indicate that the type of treatment and economic status affect the quality of life of cancer patients. Also, according to Hanson, family health is related to religious, sociological and cultural factors of the family system.

According to Dorkim, the family is part of a society and knowing it requires knowing the whole society. The beliefs of each community shape the solutions that the family offers to a chronic or life-threatening illness. For example, a person with cancer believes in acupuncture instead of the treatment recommended by doctors. According to Friedman, social change has a huge impact on family life. Economic and Belief Trends of the Family Technological, demographic, political and socio-cultural developments are important factors that affect the family. Therefore, according to the above and the differences between different societies, the results of studies conducted in other countries about the family cannot be generalized to Iran because each family is a secret and unique and like a mirror of the main elements It encompasses society and is a reflection of social unrest. It is also important to note that the existence of family ties and ties among Iranians has deep roots. Biman believes that in Iran, the obligations related to the sincere relationship and equality in the institution of the family are crystallized and continued in the best way.

In a study conducted by Ghanbari in 2009 in Iran with the aim of determining the priorities of cancer nursing research, it was found that according to cancer nurses, the issue of psychological and social effects of cancer diagnosis on the family is among the 10 research priorities with a frequency distribution of 94.4 Percentage has the highest research priority. However, similar studies conducted in European and American countries showed different results. Prioritizing nursing research topics for cancer patients in different countries can be a reflection of the philosophy and health care system of those countries.

For example, the difference in the priority of nursing research in European and American countries is related to the difference in the evolution of cancer nursing research in these countries. According to these results, in recent years, there is a need to determine national and regional strategies. When working with a family, the health nurse should consider not only the differences in the health needs of families, but also the differences in the resources available to families in different communities and the different priorities and needs of families in different communities.

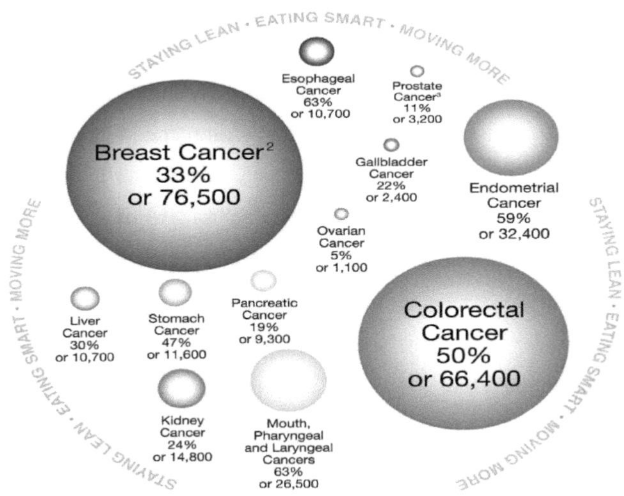

Figure 3. Cancer Prevention with a Healthful Lifestyle

Based on the above and the importance of the family in community health studies, as well as the researcher's experiences as a cancer nurse in working with cancer patients and their families, which in most cases witness obvious disorders in the relationships of patients' family members as separation, child dropout and ... and also the difference in the impact of cancer on the family due to cultural and socio-economic differences of families in different communities and the lack of basic information about the impact of cancer on indigenous families, we decided to improve family functioning in families. Let's investigate that one of the couples has cancer.

Ways to reduce your cancer risk

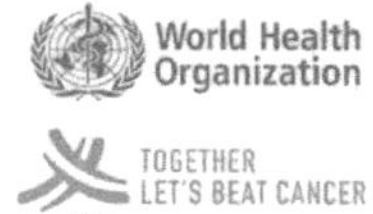

Do not smoke or use any form of tobacco

Make your home **smoke-free**

Avoid too much sun, use **sun protection**

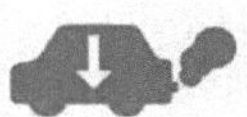
Reduce indoor and outdoor **air pollution**

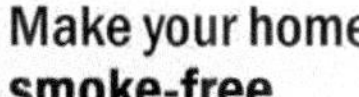
Enjoy a **healthy diet**

Be **physically active**

Breastfeeding reduces the mother's cancer risk

Limit alcohol intake

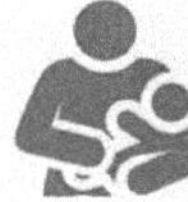
Vaccinate your children against Hepatitis B and HPV

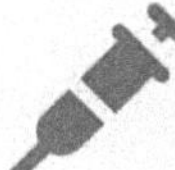
Take part in organized **cancer screening programmes**

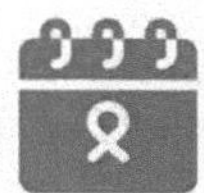

Figure 4. Lifestyle To Cut Cancer Risk

Definition of words

Family

Theoretical definition

It is a group of people who interact with each other as husband, wife, mother, father, brother and sister through marriage, inbreeding or adoption (as children), create a common culture and live in a certain unit. The family is defined as a system of two or more individuals joined by blood or emotional connections.

Practical definition

A family is a group of legally married people of the opposite sex who live in the same house, may have children, and one of the couples is diagnosed with cancer by an oncologist.

Couples

Theoretical definition

Couples are two people who are married.

Practical definition

The couple in this study refers to a man and a woman who are legally married to each other, live in the same house, have been married for more than a year, and may have children.

Cancer

Theoretical definition

It is a pathogenic process that causes abnormal proliferation of cells and ignores growth-regulating signals in the environment around the cells.

Family function

Theoretical definition

Family function means the ability of the family to adapt to changes made during life, conflict resolution, solidarity between members, implementation of the rules governing this institution, with the aim of maintaining the entire family system.

Practical definition

Family performance was measured with the standard FAD family measurement tool which has 7 items.

Understand

Theoretical definition

Perception is a process that refers to a person's awareness of what is being presented through the sensory organs. Perception is not direct awareness of sensory apparatus data, as this data reassembles under the influence of cognitive processes and infer patterns. Perception may be taken into account or ignored, but it cannot be cut off at will.

Perception is the experience of conscious sensory perception, which is a process of constant change that converts the brain's electrical signals into sensory experiences. Perception usually leads to action.

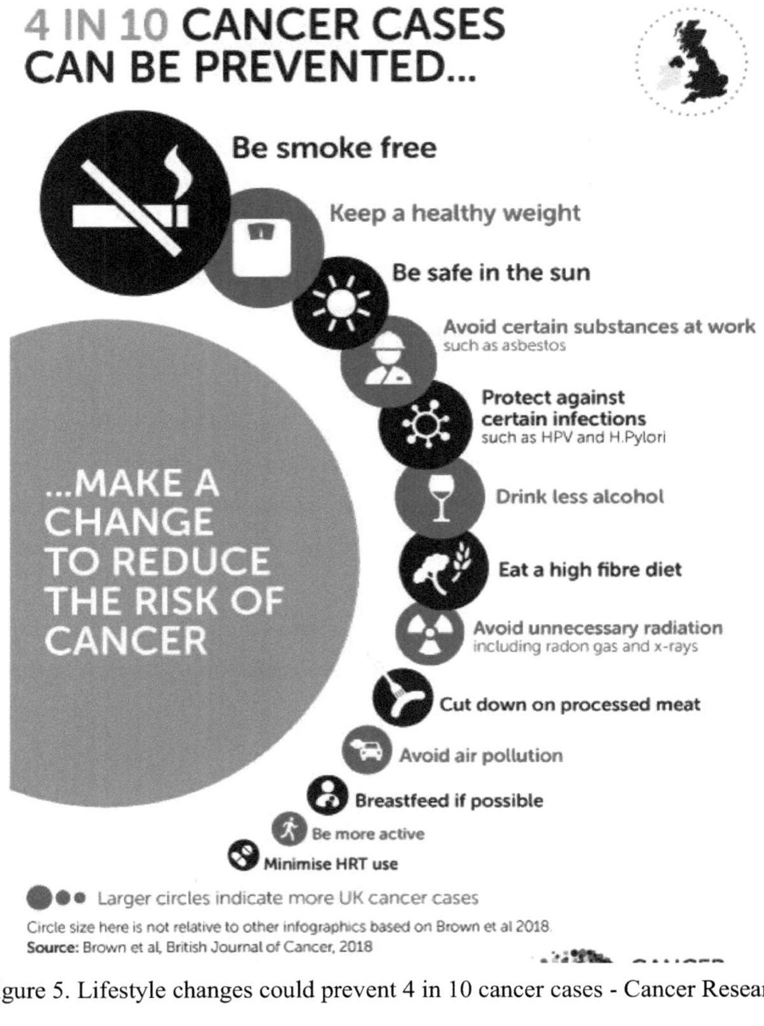

Figure 5. Lifestyle changes could prevent 4 in 10 cancer cases - Cancer Research UK

Chapter II

What is cancer?

Cancer is a pathogenic process that causes abnormal cell proliferation and ignores growth-regulating signals around the cells. Cancer is not an independent disease with a single cause, but includes a separate set of diseases that have different causes, manifestations, treatments and prognoses. Cancer is actually a disease of cells, not organs. Every malignancy starts with a cell or group of cells that are inherently normal but have changed in some way. The end result of this change is the loss of all or part of the normal properties and the manifestation of abnormal properties in the cells. The change that occurs affects the appearance of the cell and its membrane surface and its growth characteristics.

Pathophysiology of the malignant process: Cancer is a pathogenic process that begins when the DNA of a normal cell changes due to a genetic mutation.

This abnormal cell forms a clone and begins to multiply abnormally, regardless of the growth-regulating messages or signals around the cell. The cells then find invasive features and changes in the surrounding tissue occur. The cells penetrate the lymphatic and blood vessels through these tissues, and the blood and lymph vessels, in turn, carry these cells to other areas of the body. This phenomenon is called metastasis (spread of cancer to other areas of the body).

Etiology

Factors or factors that are somehow involved in the process of carcinogenesis include viruses and bacteria, physical factors, chemical factors, genetic or familial factors, dietary factors and hormonal factors.

Viruses and bacteria: It is difficult to identify the viruses that cause cancer in humans, because it is difficult to separate viruses. Only in the case of certain cancers that present as a group can the presence of infectious causes be considered or suspected. Viruses are believed to integrate with the genetic structure of the cell, resulting in the next generation of the same cell being altered or possibly cancerous.

Physical factors: The most important physical factors associated with carcinogenesis are: exposure to sunlight or radiation, chronic irritation or inflammation, and tobacco use.

Chemical agents: About 75% of all cancers are thought to be related to the environment. Tobacco smoke is the deadliest chemical carcinogen, accounting for at least 30% of cancer deaths.

The most dangerous chemical agents are substances that reveal their toxic effects by altering the structure of DNA, and do so on areas of the body that are far from the area of chemical contact. In this regard, the liver, lungs and kidneys are among the organ systems that are most affected by these cases, perhaps due to their role in detoxification of chemicals.

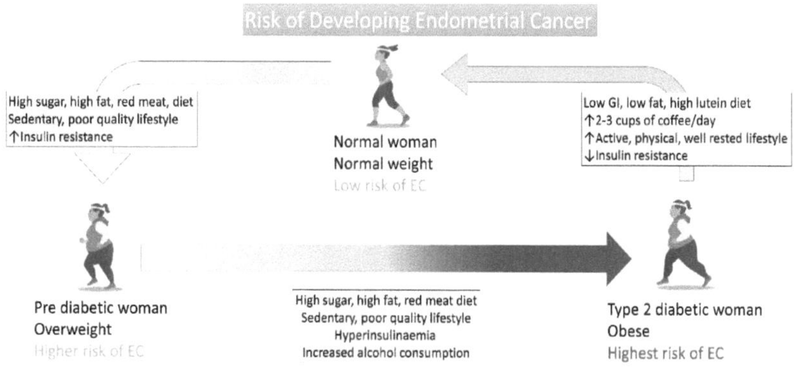

Figure 6. Narrative Review of the Role of Diet and Lifestyle Factors

Genetic and familial factors: It has been found that almost any type of cancer can occur in families, the cause of which should be attributed to the genetic context of common environments, cultural factors and lifestyle, sometimes the occurrence of cancer in families is accidental and It is incidental and does not depend on a specific factor.

Genetic factors also play a role in the development of cancer cells. The presence of extra chromosomes, the very small number of chromosomes, and the displacement of chromosomes with abnormal chromosomal patterns are associated with cancer. In approximately 5% of childhood and adult cancers, there is a family orientation.

Nutritional factors: These factors are associated with environmental cancers. Foods can be divided into 3 types: carcinogen, carcinogenic aid, and preventive (protective). Lack of preventive foods in the diet for a long time and the presence of carcinogenic foods and carcinogenic aids increase the risk of cancer. Fats, alcohol, smoked meats and salty salts, foods high in nitrate and nitrite, and high-calorie diets are some of the factors that are associated with a higher risk of cancer.

Hormonal factors: Disorders in hormonal balance, which are either due to the production of hormones by the body itself (androgen) or the consumption of external hormones (exogenous), can promote tumor growth.

In general, the word "cancer" is used like the term "umbrella" to cover a large group of diseases (more than 200 types of diseases) that, although they have different side effects, treatment and prognosis, in every part of the body. When created, they create common features. The downside of the word "cancer" is that it usually has negative connotations for people. So answering the question "What is cancer?" it is difficult. One way to understand cancer is to know how it occurs in the population. Therefore, this section briefly describes the epidemiology of cancer.

Epidemiology

Cancer is a common disease that 1 in 3 people will experience at some point in their lives.

Although cancer can affect all age groups, it is more common in people over the age of 65. In general, men are more likely than women to get cancer, and more than half of all cancers occur in developing countries. In most developing countries, cancer is the second leading cause of death after cardiovascular disease. Of course, in Iran it is the third reason.

Every year, 7.5 million new cases are added to the cancer statistics in the world. In the UK alone, 25,000 people are diagnosed with cancer each year. The American Cancer Society estimates the number of new cases of cancer and cancer deaths each year. In 2012, it was predicted that in 2014 there would be 1665,540 new cases of cancer and 585,720 deaths due to cancer in the United States, which shows an increase of 1.8% in men and an increase of 1.4% in women. To cancer in the United States. However, overall cancer mortality in 2009 decreased by 20% compared to 1991, when the highest death rate was reported that year.

In Iran, as a developing country, cancer is the third leading cause of death after heart disease, accidents and other phenomena. According to the results of Mousavi's study in 2009, the annual incidence of cancer among Iranian men and women is 98 and 110 per 100,000, respectively. According to the World Health Organization, the number of cancer deaths worldwide will increase by 45% from 2007 to 2030 (from 7.9 million to 11.5 million deaths). Therefore, cancer causes a huge burden of disease. In Iran, 3,000 people die every year due to cancer. It is reported that 50% of the most common cancers in Iran are related to the gastrointestinal tract, and among the cancers of the gastrointestinal tract, colon cancer. It has the highest incidence of gastric cancer. This cancer ranks third in women and fifth in men. The prevalence of this disease in the country is increasing in both sexes and is considered as one of the most important cancers that has a high mortality rate. Also, since most cancers occur in the elderly and Iran has a relatively young population, with increasing life expectancy, it is expected that in the near future the incidence and mortality of this deadly disease in the country will increase rapidly. Therefore, it is necessary to pay attention to the importance of fighting this deadly disease and the existence of a cancer control program in the country.

Impact of cancer on the individual

A diagnosis of cancer can cause shock and anger in patients, disrupting their normal lives. This shock initially leads to deep feelings of disbelief and in some cases an obvious denial of the disease. These reactions are often characterized by acute fear and stress and are likened to "fever" or "mental infection." Adaptation to the diagnosis of cancer is influenced by a number of factors, including how the definitive diagnosis of cancer is transmitted to the individual, individual opinions about the disease, delay in diagnosis, individual personality, and adaptation practices that the individual uses in crisis situations. Patients with cancer typically experience a range of symptoms, including two types of physical and mental disorders. Immediately after diagnosis, anxiety and other mood disorders may develop in the individual, which change over time and in response to diagnosis, recurrence and improvement of the disease.

This disease is unique in terms of the feeling of helplessness and deep fear that it creates in a person. There is no doubt that the diagnosis of life-threatening diseases such as cancer has several effects on a person's quality of life. Cancer is not just an event with a definite end, but an ambiguous permanent situation characterized by the delayed effects of illness, treatment, and related psychological issues.

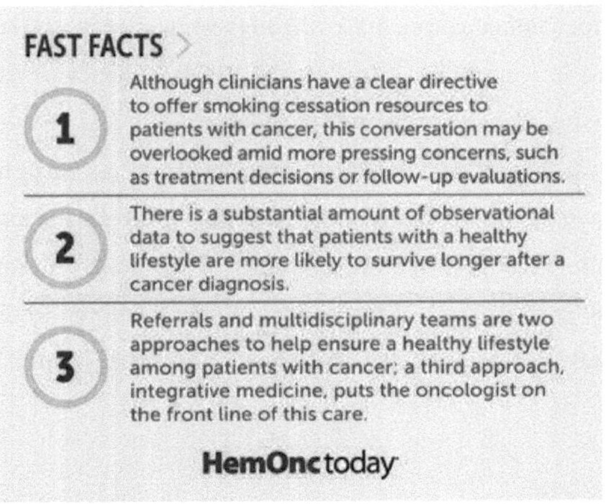

Figure 7. Making lifestyle changes 'part of the cancer treatment conversation'

The impact of cancer on the family

Numerous studies have confirmed the effect of cancer on the physical, social and psychological well-being of the family. It is widely accepted that the fight against cancer is a family affair. Not only the patient, but also everyone who loves him or her, is dealing with the consequences of illness and treatment, which may include disruption of daily life, anxiety, depression, worry about cancer recurrence, fear of losing the affected person. And death. The news of cancer diagnosis in a spouse, friend or relative can cause severe emotional distress in the form of sadness, depression, anxiety or anger. Also, daily functioning can be altered or disrupted. This change is due to weight loss, fatigue or insomnia. This experience occurs not only for the person with cancer, but also for the patient's family members throughout the course of the disease. A sense of threat of losing a person due to cancer develops in the family, which triggers a sense of sadness in the family, which in turn disrupts the organization and description of feelings, activities, values, and priorities.

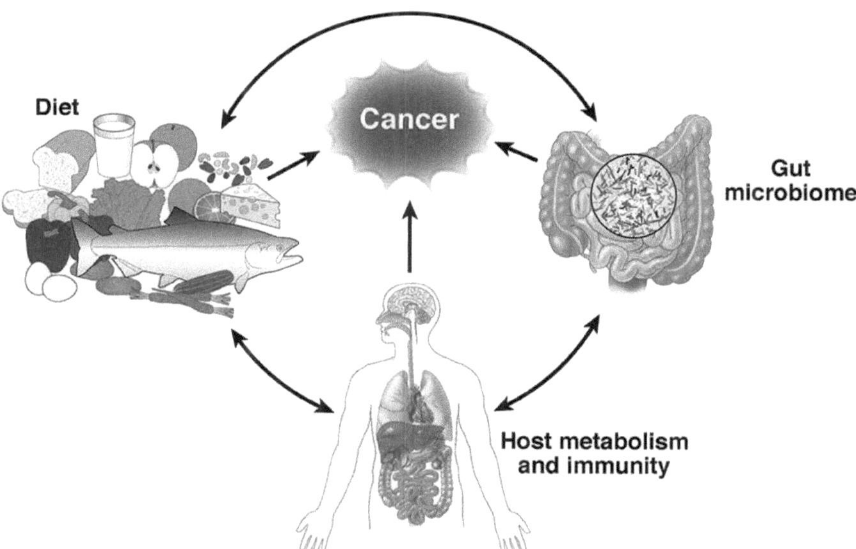

Figure 8. Diet, Lifestyle, Gut Microbiome, and Cancer Prevention and Treatment

Therefore, the feeling of sadness can be not only due to the loss of a person, but also due to the loss of a part of life experiences. Family life may change dramatically as a result of a cancer diagnosis, and family members may take on new tasks in addition to their usual life tasks.

Also, important aspects of family life may be flawed. For example, family vacations are planned for a short period of time, or the family may face financial difficulties because most of the family income is spent on cancer treatment, and as a result, the family may even have to sell to pay for treatment. There are also changes in daily life plans that are less obvious, such as feelings of uncertainty and ambiguity about plans and hopes for the future. Also, family members live in a state of insecurity, insecurity, and possible fear that may become a reality, preparing themselves for a horrible life without the person they love.

Severe illness can disrupt family life, impair family functioning, damage or deform resources, and burden the caregiver. The family's ability to cope with the crisis depends on their resources. Family resources, including:

Social resources: A strong social network that can include a spouse, child, parents, siblings, friends, and more.

Cultural resources: Cultural values that can affect a family or individual's ability to care for a patient and cope with stress.

Religious sources: including religious beliefs, religious customs.

Educational resources: The level of formal education that a person receives and allows him or her to understand the patient's condition and provide appropriate care.

Medical resources: includes access to medical facilities and equipment that assist caregivers.

The effect of cancer on couples' relationships

Numerous studies have shown that cancer has a significant impact on spouses, and it is very important to focus more on spouses in examining family members of people with cancer. Information on non-medical issues, such as coping with cancer or the impact of cancer on relationships, is more likely to be overlooked in patients' spouses and family members than medical information. May be experienced. The reason for this feeling is that when hearing the news of a cancer diagnosis, the first thought that comes to patients' spouses is that the person they love is on the verge of death. In fact, spouses are more afraid of death than patients themselves. Also, studies on the wives of women with breast cancer have shown that breast cancer is a disease of couples and for the wives of those patients, it is extremely stressful. Thus, cancer has a significant effect on the patient and his spouse in terms of body image, gender and their relationship. Husbands fear for their future, the future of their children, and the progression and recurrence of cancer during the active period of cancer. The amount of stress and tension that men and women experience when their husbands are infected. Studies have shown that women receive as much stress as their wives when their husbands do get cancer. But the amount of stress that men get when they get cancer is greater than when their wives get it.

Therefore, women are more affected by their husbands' illness than men. Researchers have cited two reasons for this difference: first, women are more stressed because they spend more time on care tasks, and second, men caring for a sick spouse is more satisfying for men than women. Slow and raises their self-esteem. Traditionally, women have been viewed as family caregivers. As a result, they may set high standards for their caring role and have high expectations of themselves. Men, on the other hand, feel good about themselves because the role they play when their wives are ill being not normally expected of them. A number of studies on couples also show that couples' relationships when one of them has cancer, has become more positive, and cancer has improved their quality of life and serves as an opportunity to improve the couple's relationship and bring them closer together.

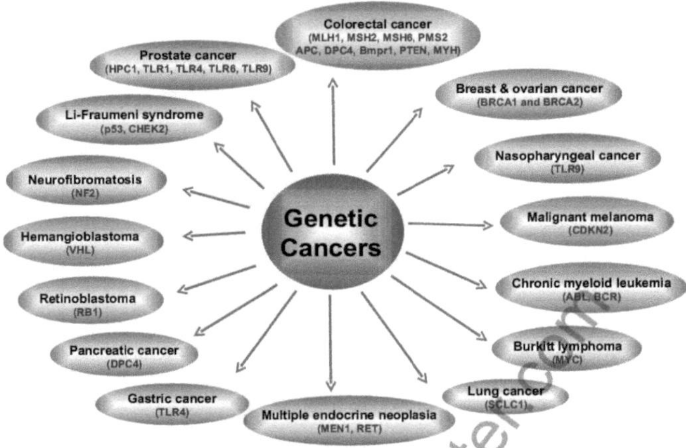

Figure 9. Cancer is a Preventable Disease that Requires Major Lifestyle Changes

The effect of parental cancer on children

When parents are diagnosed with cancer, their children receive considerable stress. Because children have little information about the nature of this disease. Increasing children's responsibilities and decreasing their social activity are considered as the most significant changes in children's lives. The presence of life-threatening disease in parents causes disruption in the natural process of the family and stress in its members, especially children, and causes physical, psychological and social problems in the child, which will cause a shaky personality structure in adulthood. Many researchers agree that children whose parents have a chronic illness are at risk for behavioral problems. Due to the high rate of chronic illness, the number of children at risk for depression, anxiety and psychological symptoms is high.

Therefore, caregivers should be aware of these problems for interventions and keep in mind that children from young families, single parents, low-income families, and parents with longer periods of illness need more support. Therefore, rapid identification of children at risk after parents become ill is the most important step to prevent behavioral problems in children. Because medical staff often pay attention to the patient's parent and spouse, and children are marginalized. While these same children may be lifelong caregivers of their sick parents, even fathers whose spouses have cancer sometimes do not recognize their children's grief and interpret some of their reactions as "child abuse". While children are often aware of their father's emotional state and try to protect him.

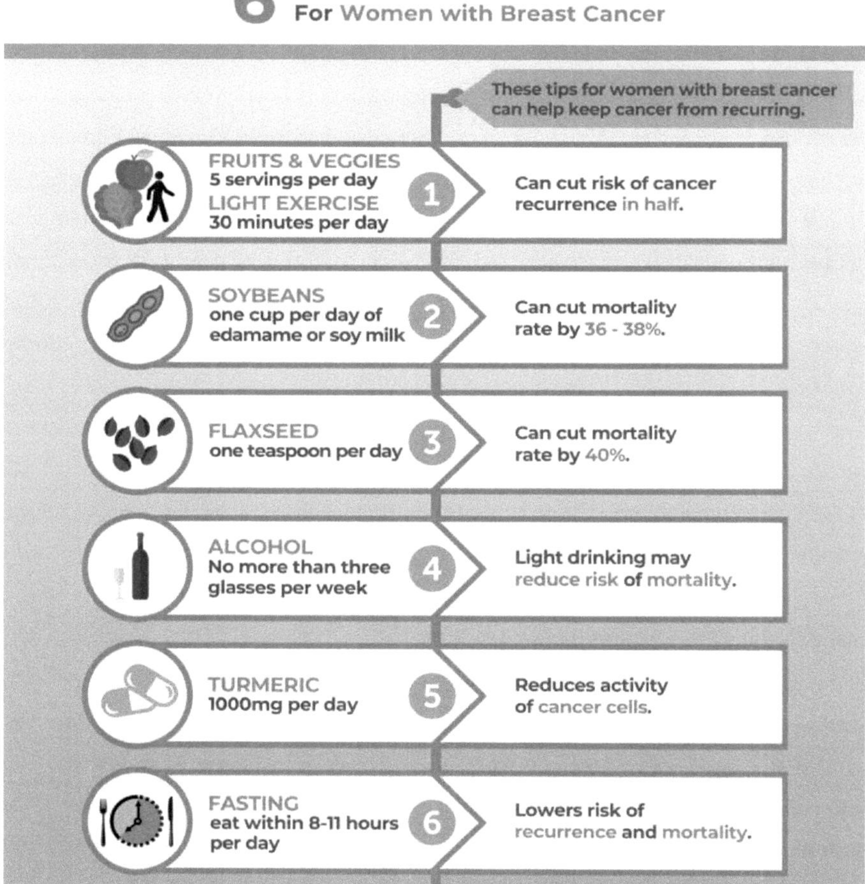

Figure 10. Reducing Your Breast Cancer Risk: 6 Healthy Lifestyle Tips for Women

The physical condition of cancer patients is associated with severe role dysfunction and consequent contact with their children. When sick parents are less able to care for family members, children have to face new tasks. Also, research shows that children of parents with cancer who have a bachelor's degree or higher are at lower risk of developing mental health problems than children of parents with lower education, and the proportion of children with mental health problems in mothers with similar cancers This ratio is affected in fathers. In contrast, some researchers believe that the children of affected parents do not have serious psychological or social problems compared to the control group and are at low risk of psychological problems. Female children seem to be more affected by the negative effects of parental illness.

France believes that the effects of cancer on children should not be pathological because although there is tension and confusion in children, parental cancer is an unusual transition in the life of children rather than a pathological process! For this reason, interventions should be directed towards programs that can shape the child's perspective when parents have cancer so that children can cope with this stage of their lives and adapt. In other words, instead of changing the course of the river, accept it and organize it with the rocks in the course of the river. Before addressing the concept of family functioning, we first need to consider the concept of family and its importance in community health studies.

The concept of family and its importance

The Latin word Family is derived from the word "Familia" meaning the servants of a family, which includes two or more people who are related by blood or marriage. In Sanskrit, family is referred to as dhman, meaning place of residence. Most cultures and languages define the family as related.

From the beginning of human existence on the planet, men and women have always lived together by forming a center called the family, raising children in their laps and leaving this world. The most natural form of the family is that nothing but death can break the marriage bond. The main elements of a family are a woman and a man who are married to each other according to their social customs and then a child or children are added to them.

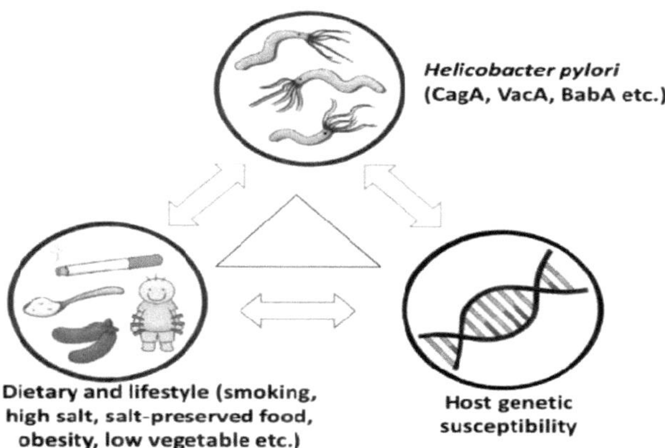

Figure 11. Risk factors of gastric cancer. Interaction of dietary and lifestyle

The family is one of the first social institutions that has a specific structure that is affected by social changes and developments. The family is the smallest unit of society, this social unit is the source of human emotions and the center of the most intimate interpersonal relationships and interactions.

The importance of the family is such that the health and growth of any society depends on the health and growth of the family. The family is one of the most common social organizations and is formed on the basis of marriage between at least two opposite sexes, in which real and documented blood relations can be seen. The family usually has a kind of spatial commonality and is responsible for various personal, physical, economic, and educational functions. The family is a social symbol and like a mirror contains the main elements of society and is a reflection of social disorders. In addition, the family is one of the most important factors affecting society. No society can ever be healthy unless it has healthy families.

The family is the closest unit of life to man. The vast majority of human beings are born into a family and take the first vital steps in it. The vast majority of people also build a family and spend their whole lives in it. Therefore, recognizing this social unit will be difficult due to its proximity to humans.

Family is defined in different ways. The difference in the definition of family depends on the descriptive theoretical background. For example, authors who support interactionist theories view the family as an arena for the interaction of characters, thus, in their definition of the family, they emphasize the characteristics of the interactive dynamics of the family.

The authors, who support the view of general systems, define the family as a small arm social system that consists of interdependent components and is influenced by its internal structure and external environment. In this study, the family is examined under the influence of a recent perspective. Because understanding the overall functioning of the family requires understanding the performance of the individual family members, the functioning of the family as a unit, and the relationship between the family and society, the theory of family systems, derived from general systems theory, seems to be a the theory is useful for understanding different levels of family functioning. Also, understanding the family as a system helps to identify the cause of the problem and stress in the family and allows the therapist or family counselor to better identify the goals and methods of treatment.

Why is working with family so important when planning for health care?

Community health researchers have found that the family is the core of health care because the family is a fundamental unit that significantly influences the development of individuals, so that it may determine the success or failure of a person's life. Slowly The two main goals of any family are to meet the needs of the community of which the family is a part and to meet the needs of the family members themselves.

The family is a vital resource for providing effective health care for individuals. The following reasons highlight the importance of focusing on the family unit in providing health care:

1- The family is a vital resource for providing health care to individuals and families. When a family focuses on providing health care to its members, the effectiveness of care increases. Also, one of the goals of primary health care is to increase the level of well-being of the family, which in the next levels, increases the well-being of family members.

2- In the family unit, any defective function (illness, injury, separation, etc.) that affects a family member, in various ways, as well as the family unit as a whole, is affected. Give. Because the family is an interconnected network.

3- There is a strong interrelationship between the family and the health status of its members that the role of the family in any form of health care of each family member from the stage of health promotion to the stage of rehabilitation is very decisive.

4- Diagnosis is another good reason to provide family-centered health care. Checking for a member's health problem may lead to coverage for illness or risk factors for other family members, which usually happens when a family visit has a chronic health problem. A family-centered nurse often works with a family member to reach out to other members.

5- Another way to be able to gain a clear and comprehensive understanding of individuals and their performance is to examine them in the context of the family.

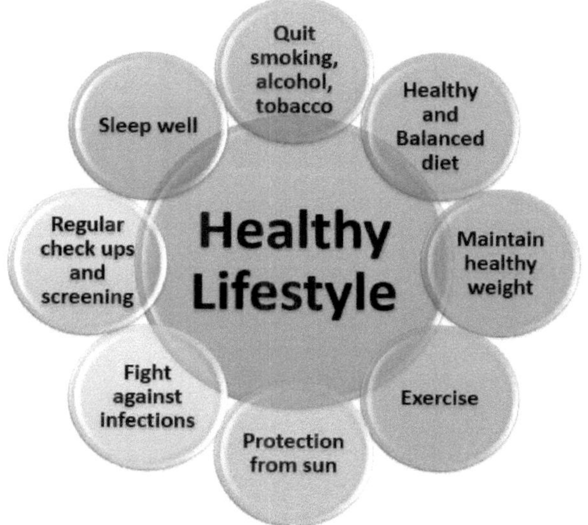

Figure 12. Lifestyle Modifications to Prevent Cancer

Sickness / health status of the family and its members interact with each other. An illness in the family affects the whole family and its interactions. On the other hand, the family also affects the health / illness of the members. Families tend to react to the health problems of family members and diagnose their health problems. Research in the field of family health shows that families have a powerful effect on the physical health of their members.

On the other hand, the family tends to be involved in deciding on treatment procedures at every stage of illness and health of family members, from health promotion and prevention strategies to diagnosis, treatment and recovery. The process of "becoming ill" and receiving health services It requires a series of decisions and events that require the interactions of a number of people, including family, friends, and health care providers. However, the role that the family plays in this process at all times depends on the health of the individual, the type of health problem (such as whether the problem is acute or chronic), and the degree of family involvement.

The 6 stages of health / illness and family interaction are:

1- Family efforts to promote health;
2- Assessing the family of the symptoms of the disease;
3- Seeking care;
4- Obtaining care;
5- Acute responses to the disease by the patient and family;
6- Adaptation to the disease and recovery.

The presence of a chronic and serious illness in a family member usually has a profound effect on the family system, especially on the structure of the individual role and the performance of family functions. Families are the first caregivers of chronic diseases. When each of the individual situations is serious and the family member is a pivotal and important person in family functioning, the impact on family functioning is felt a little more.

Family function

Family functioning is generally described as a consequence of family structure. Some authors consider the term "performance" to mean "achievement" or "result", therefore, they consider family performance as what the family does.

Family function means the ability of the family to adapt to changes made during life, conflict resolution, solidarity between members, implementation of the rules governing this institution, with the aim of maintaining the entire family system. Family functioning includes behaviors and activities performed by family members to maintain the family and meet the needs of the family and members.

wright and Lehy have divided the family performance survey into two parts: instrumental performance and expressive performance. Instrumental function refers to daily life activities such as absorption and excretion, sleep, rest, insulin intake, and so on.

The second type of family performance review is the performance or emotional and psychological aspects of the family, which include:

Emotional communication: such as whether the family is able to express the amount of emotions including anger, happiness and sadness?

Verbal and non-verbal communication: Verbal communication focuses on the meaning of words and non-verbal communication is a type of communication that includes sounds, gestures, eye contact, touch or silence. An example of non-verbal communication is that, for example, when the wife speaks, the husband stares out the window!

Problem solving goes back to how the family solves the problem. Who identifies the problem? What kind of problems have been identified? What patterns have been used to solve the problem?

Roles go back to established patterns of behavior. Roles may be created, assigned, and negotiated in the family. This allows family members to take on a role. Formal roles in the family may be influenced by religion, culture, and other belief systems.

In the following, the dimensions of family representation performance are described according to the McMaster model:

To understand the structure, organization, and patterns of family interaction, this model examines and formulates 6 aspects of life, including problem solving, communication, roles, emotional responsiveness, emotional cohesion, and behavior control. These are aspects of clinical practice that are thought to be useful in the clinic.

1- Problem solving

Problem solving is defined as the family's ability to solve problems that maintain effective family functioning. Sanaei also refers to this dimension as the family's ability to solve problems in such a way that effective interactions continue in the family. The family problem is considered as an issue that the family is hesitant to find a solution to, and this problem threatens the integrity and functional capacity of the family. Problems can be perceptually divided into instrumental problems and emotional problems. Instrumental problems are everyday problems, such as managing money or making decisions about where to live, and emotional problems are those that are related to emotional experiences.

2- Communications

The dimension of communication is thought of as how information changes in the family and according to the dual definition of communication, i.e. how the family exchanges information within itself. Communication is a self-regulatory, purposeful and organized process in the family. The primary task of the family is to communicate, because communication promotes growth and development, increases self-confidence and socialization of family members.

In the family, the focus is more on verbal communication. Non-verbal aspects of communication in the family, despite their importance, are out of the pattern because they are difficult to measure for research purposes. The communication dimension, like the problem-solving dimension, can be divided into emotional and instrumental domains, which can have an overlap between these two domains. In the McMaster model, communication is used as a general term to describe healthy behaviors in the family.

Four communication methods include

1- Clear and direct communication: In this type of communication, both the goal and the message are clear.

2- Clear and indirect communication

3- Direct and covered (hidden)

4- Indirect and covered

It should be noted that in healthy families, family communication in both emotional and instrumental areas is direct and clear.

Communication and problem solving are the most important components of the family functioning process that may facilitate the assignment and retention of roles. Milani also considers effective communication as the cornerstone of a healthy and successful family and states that "communication is essential for meeting the needs of members, proper and effective functioning and achieving family goals".

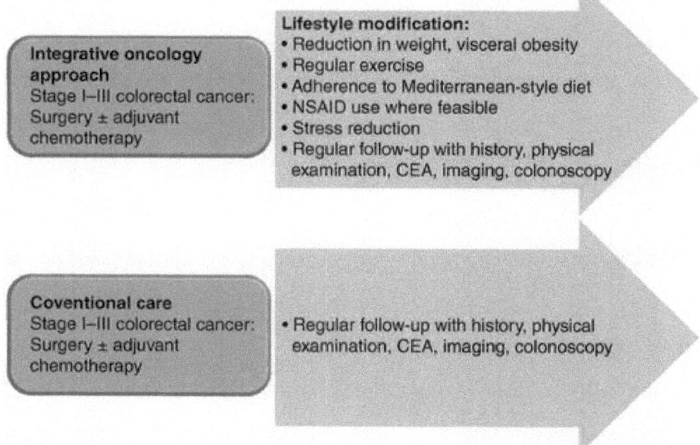

Figure 13. Lifestyle modification in colorectal cancer patients: an integrative oncology approach

3- Roles

Repetitive patterns of behaviors through which family members realize family reactions. Families have to perform some repetitive behaviors to maintain the effectiveness of the family system. Roles are divided into 3 instrumental areas, expressive and a combination of these two. 5 essential family functions include:

1- Providing resources: The roles that fall into this area are mostly tools. Such as providing food, clothing and shelter for the family

2- Training and support: Roles in this field are considered as emotional performance, which includes providing comfort, security, confidence and support to members.

3- Sexual satisfaction: It is one of the emotional functions, it is very important for couples to feel satisfied with sexual intercourse.

4- Personality development: Roles in this area are both emotional and instrumental, which include tasks related to the development of the child and the acquisition of life skills, such as helping the child to start school, or helping the teenager to take up a profession.

5- Survival and management of the family system: This area, like paragraph 4, includes several types of functions that include the techniques and measures needed to establish current standards in the family.

In the McMaster model, the best performing families are those in which each member has roles and is responsible for performing tasks related to that particular role.

4- Emotional responsiveness

The degree and quality of interest and concern of family members towards each other. Emotional responsiveness is thought of as the family's ability to respond to stimuli with the appropriate quality and quantity of emotions. In discussing quality, two questions arise, first, do family members respond to a wide range of emotions experienced in a person's emotional life? Second, are the emotions experienced compatible with the stimuli of each situation? Limited expression of emotional pain is allowed.

5- Emotional mixing

It refers to the level of participation and cooperation of family members. The emotional dimension is considered as the amount of value that each family as a whole give to the activities and interests of family members. The focus is on how much and in what way family members are interested in each other's values and engage themselves. Six types of emotional intercourse have been identified in families, ranging from complete absence of intercourse to extensive intercourse.

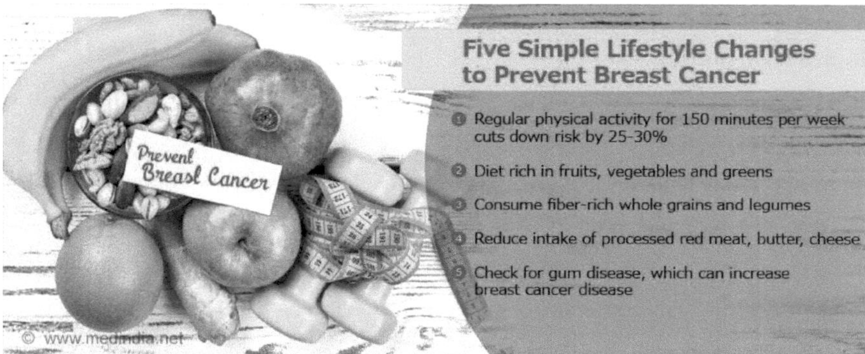

Figure 14. Five Simple Lifestyle Changes To Prevent Breast Cancer

The following are six types of intercourse:

1- Lack of intercourse: Family members show no interest in each other and live only in one place.

2- Intercourse without emotions: In this type, there is little interest, but members invest a little of their emotions in interaction with another. That is, the investment of feelings and emotions for others is made when requested, and to a very small extent.

3- Narcissistic or narcissistic intercourse: Others have no special place in the person.

4- Compassionate intercourse: Family members show real emotional concern for each other's interests.

5- Extreme intercourse: This type of intercourse is characterized by showing excessive interfering behaviors and excessive support of members to each other.

6- Cohabiting intercourse: Emotional intercourse is so intense that the existing boundaries between family members have disappeared.
Compassionate companionship is the most effective and healthiest type of intercourse. Be recognized as malfunctioning.

6- Behavior control

It is a model that the family adopts to manage behavior in three situations: physical, psychological-biological and social. First, there are situations of physical danger in which the family monitors and controls the behavior of its members. Second, it satisfies the psycho-biological needs of its members such as eating, drinking, sleeping, and sexual needs in a variety of situations, and ultimately there are situations that govern interpersonal socialization behavior in family members and those outside the family. It is important to consider the behavior of all family members in each situation. In the series of surveys, the appropriateness of family rules and standards, the age and circumstances of those involved should be considered. Families set the standard for their acceptable behaviors as well as the degree of freedom they give to those standards. The nature of these standards and the degree of freedom of action for acceptable behaviors is called the degree of behavior control in the family.

This dimension shows both the standards and expectations of parents' behavior towards their children and the standards of children's behavior towards each other. There are four ways to control behavior:

Rigid Behavior Control: Family rules include strict standards that allow members little flexibility in any situation.

Flexible Behavior Control: Standards and rules are reasonable in the eyes of family members and there is opportunity for negotiation and change.

Controlling unruly behavior: There is no standard in the family.

Irregular Behavior Control: In this type of behavior control, the family tends to have an unpredictable and random pattern between a rigid, flexible, and restrained pattern. Family members do not know which standards to apply to what extent and when. Flexible behavior control is the most efficient form and irregular type is the most ineffective type of behavior control.

Optimal family performance

Higher-performing families are referred to in community health texts as healthy families, but it should be noted that attempts to define a "normal" or "healthy" family, especially for researchers who use the family as a system of interaction. With each other and with other subsystems (cultural, political, economic, biological, social) define, it is a futile endeavor. Because "normal" often means not having any particular problem that cannot apply to the family, it is difficult to label the family "healthy" or "unhealthy". According to Lancaster, labeling families as "unhealthy" or "poorly performing" does not allow families to change or intervene in nursing to meet their needs. Families are not all good or all bad. Therefore, nurses need to evaluate family behavior in the range of different needs of each family in order to properly assess the family and pay attention to the fact that all families have strengths and weaknesses.

Given the problems mentioned, a common way to describe the optimal performance of the family is to use statistical concepts such as the average that the family is measured based on the scores obtained from the samples, and therefore if the selected sample represents the community, family characteristics Obtained from that community that this method of describing family functioning is used in the McMaster model.

As long as the family seems "normal", it can be helpful to be aware of the concept of a well-functioning family. Many therapists like to solve other problems in addition to the problem raised by the family. To this end, Krishner and Krishner (1986) have developed the "optimal family process" model, which is very valuable. In describing the optimal functioning of the family, the two consider marriage interactions, educational interactions, and independent interactions, and examine the individual actions of family members in their activities, whether professional, educational, social, or recreational. If the marital relationship is weak, the foundations needed for the family to be successful and desirable will be shaky or at least weak. It is difficult for a couple who are not compatible with each other to be good parents. Families have very different compositions, and healthy family action can take many forms. Exactly examining the characteristics that are important in evaluating family actions and whether they are normal or abnormal, and determining their importance, is based on the therapist's attitude and perspective. The cultural values of families and their ethnic backgrounds are also important factors.

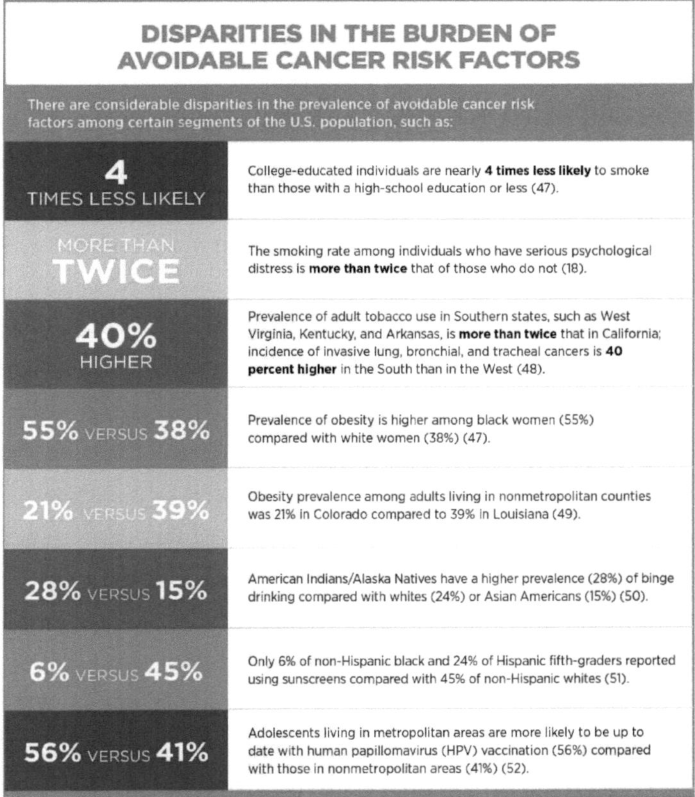

Figure 15. Preventing Cancer: Identifying Risk Factors

"Optimal family functioning" is a useful concept that is considered not only for potential problems in the family but also for determining whether the needs of the couple and their children are being met as they should be. Every family must meet both the emotional and psychological needs of its members.

Studies show that good family performance is effective in improving the quality of life and increasing the level of health of people in society, as well as reducing family problems, increasing life satisfaction, increasing life expectancy and improving life skills. By improving family functioning, children's general health can be improved and mental and physical disorders can be prevented. Good family functioning can help members cope with stress and adverse conditions. Family dysfunction confuses and worries members and causes health problems. In a family with good performance-solving problems, roles and responsibilities are clear and flexible.

As mentioned, in this study, the family has been studied under the influence of family systems theory. Because this model identifies the dimensions of family functioning that are clinically important in dealing with families.

That is, it deals with the current functioning of the family, not with the evolutionary stage of the family or its previous growth.

Therefore, before describing the McMaster model, we will first briefly explain the concepts of general systems theory and then the family systems theory that forms the theoretical framework of the McMaster model.

Systems theory and its application in family study

The theory of general systems was proposed by Van Bertalenfi (1968). He defined the system as "a set of moderating elements." In addition, he distinguished between open and closed systems. Closed systems are those that do not interact with the environment and function as a chemical or physical reaction in a closed container. Such systems follow different rules from those followed in open systems. For example, closed systems show self-analysis, tend to maximize simplicity, and reduce the situation to the simplest possible level since the beginning of the situation. Therefore, if two gases do not chemically react with each other, they will be placed in a closed container, resulting in the two not mixing completely together.

As soon as the process is complete, the system is said to be in "equilibrium". While game systems such as the family do not show analysis and the constant exchange of issues related to them is always outside the boundaries of the system. If the characteristics of the boundaries remain intact and the external environment also changes, a kind of state of stability is achieved.

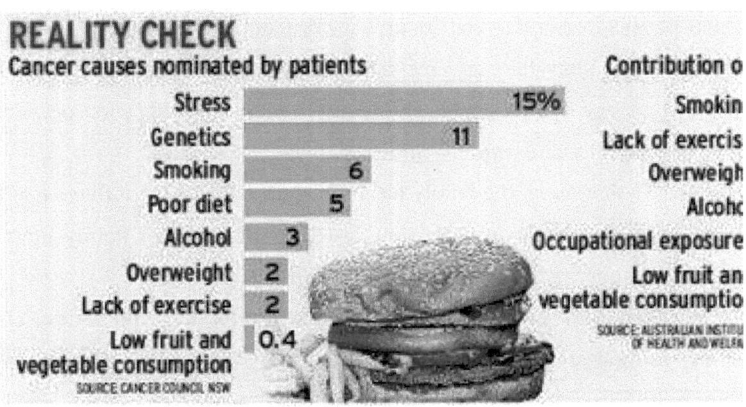

Figure 16. Cancer patients in denial over poor lifestyle choices

Of course, the environment of most open systems is resistant to change. In support of this, Zadok also states that, according to the theory of the family system, the family is a unit that operates in such a way that the moderation (homeostasis) of its interactions is maintained at all costs. In family therapy, too, the goal is to reveal the often hidden patterns that perpetuate the group's interaction and help the group understand the purpose of the pattern. Family therapists believe that a family member who has been labeled a disease is someone who is considered a family problem, should be blamed and needs help, while the therapist family aims to help the family understand the patient's symptoms. In fact, it has served the central function of the family, which is to maintain its moderation. An integral part of family system theory is the degree to which the relationship between husband and wife strongly influences the nature of the family moderation system. This concept has been expressed by one of the family therapists in a way that the couple are the architects of the family.

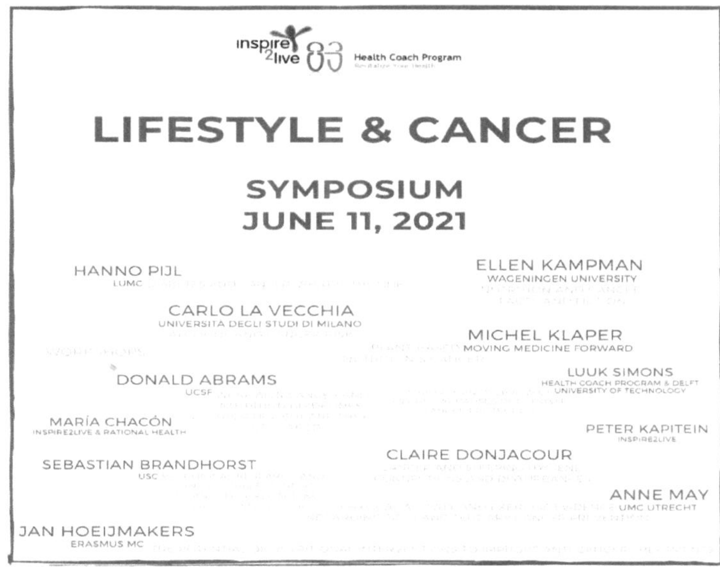

Figure 17. Lifestyle and Cancer

Sometimes there are changes in the characteristics of the borders. Therefore, the properties of open systems are likely to change or gradually become complete. The importance of systems theory in family therapy lies in the ideas and concepts it has brought to the field.

A) Families and other social groups are systems whose characteristics are more than the sum of the characteristics of their components.

B) The operation of such systems is governed by specific general laws.

C) Each system has boundaries whose characteristics are important in understanding how the system works.

D) The pervasive boundaries of the system are semi-permeable, meaning that some things can be crossed and some cannot. In addition, sometimes there are certain topics that just come in or out.

E) Family systems tend towards relative stability, not complete. In fact, their growth and development are normal, change can occur or be stimulated in different ways.

F) Communication and feedback mechanisms between system components are important in its operation.

G) Understanding events such as the behavior of family members in the form of examples such as circular causation is better than linear causation.

H) Family systems, like open systems, seem to be purposeful.

I) Systems are composed of subsystems and are in fact components of larger and more comprehensive systems.

In fact, the idea of cyclic causality versus linear causality is the basis for understanding the processes that exist in families, which of course is common to both. Linear causation describes a process that itself triggers another process. But in general, there is no idea that opening the umbrella has the slightest role in the rain. Rather, it is a case of linear causality, why event A (start of rain) is assumed to be the cause of event B (umbrella opening) but event (b) has no effect on event (a). Cyclic causality is a term that, when used, indicates a situation in which event (b) also interacts with event (a).

One of the important concepts derived from systems theory is the question of the relationship between subsystems and pervasive systems. The subsystems to which the family belongs are the open family, the village, the neighbor, the tribe, and the like, each of which in turn is part of the larger subsystems. The system that the therapist family usually focuses on is the family. But the sub-systems and usually the external systems of the families who treat them are also of interest to the therapists' families.

Each system has a boundary that distinguishes it from its surroundings. Living systems have clear and visible physical boundaries, such as the skin. But in emotional and psychological systems, boundaries are not so visible, although they are equally important. These boundaries control the inner emotional changes and bring the actions together and connect them. Some families have relatively impenetrable boundaries, completely separate from their social environment, but these boundaries are much more permeable in other families. The boundaries of all open systems are somewhat translucent, meaning that some things are allowed and some are not. This means that the integrity of the system and its distance from the environment is maintained.

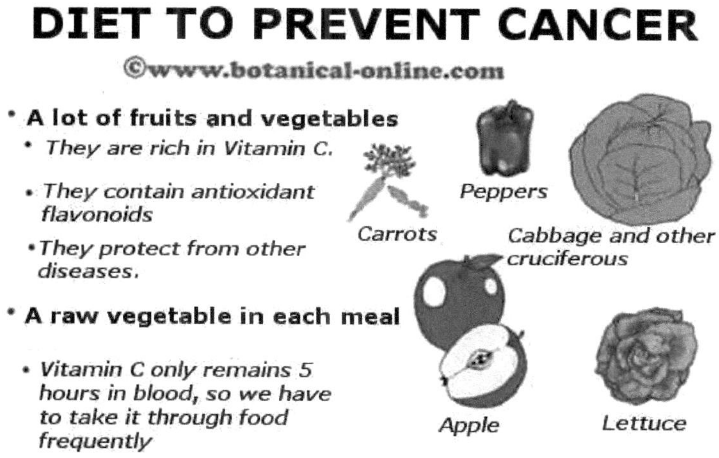

DIET TO PREVENT CANCER
©www.botanical-online.com
• A lot of fruits and vegetables
• They are rich in Vitamin C.
• They contain antioxidant flavonoids
• They protect from other diseases.
• A raw vegetable in each meal
• Vitamin C only remains 5 hours in blood, so we have to take it through food frequently
Peppers
Carrots
Cabbage and other cruciferous
Apple
Lettuce

Figure 18. Plant-based diet for cancer prevention

Family systems theory

The theory of family systems was developed by Bowden. He developed this theory to understand family functioning and the treatment of families in clinical settings. While much of this theory focuses on clinical application, including working with individuals, couples, and families, since its inception, researchers have realized the value of its application in various humanities disciplines.

Family systems theory assumes the family as an integrated system, in which all the components of the system are interconnected as well as a whole larger than the sum of its components. So that understanding the family system is possible by considering the family as a whole and the effect it has on its components and vice versa.

According to the assumptions of this theory, the family acts as an open system in interaction with the internal and external environment. The internal environment includes the subsystems of the basic family system, such as the communication subsystems of siblings, parents, children, and so on. The external environment of the family includes supra systems, i.e. the larger environmental systems of which the family is a part, such as the cultural group to which the family interacts.

Families are influenced by theories derived from physics and biology. An open system exchanges energy and matter with the environment. In contrast, the closed system is separate from its environment. The system depends on positive and negative feedback to maintain stability (homeostasis). This theory assumes:

- The family system is larger and different from the sum of its components.
- In family systems, there are different guardians and logical relationships between subsystems (mother-child) (family-community) and ...
- Boundaries in the family system can be open, closed or optional.
- Family systems are constantly changing in response to stress and changes inside and outside the environment.
- There are structural similarities in different family systems. (Isomorphism)
- A change in a part of the family system affects the whole system.

The strength of this theory is that it examines the family from both a subsystem and a supra system. This view considers the interactions within and between family subsystems as well as the interaction between the family and larger systems such as society and the world.

Also, another positive aspect of family study with systemic theory is determining the relationship between the social and cultural context of the society in which the person has grown up on the individual's behavior.

The disadvantage is that it focuses on the interaction of the family with other systems instead of individuals, which is often better focused on individuals.

McMaster model for families

The McMaster model is a comprehensive model for family examination and treatment. The main purpose of creating the McMaster model for families is to identify the basic concepts of family functioning and family therapy that, if used carefully, will allow the therapist to provide effective treatment for families. This model is designed to be generalizable and transferable to different environments, applicable to various clinical family problems, and usable for experimental research. The McMaster model is based on systems theory.

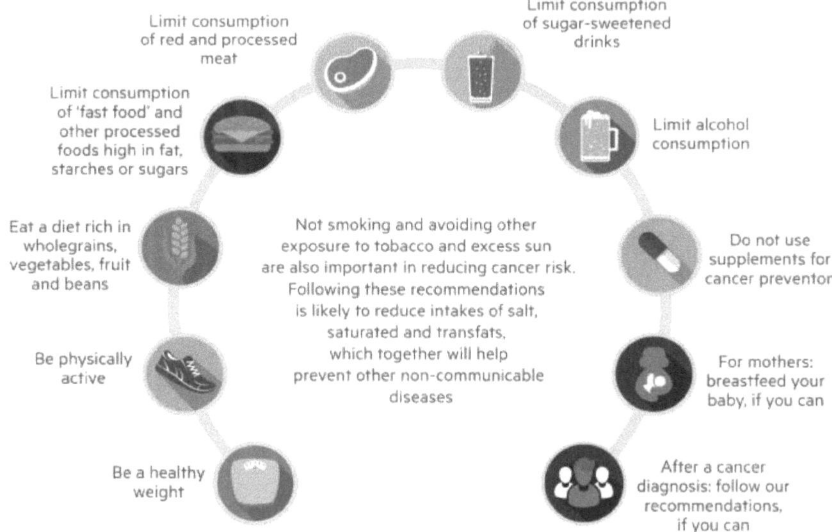

Figure 19. Spread of western lifestyle hampers battle against cancer

McMaster model assumptions for systems modeling include:

1- All parts of the family are interdependent.

2- A part of the family cannot be understood separately from other family systems.

3- A complete understanding of the family function cannot be done only with the understanding of each member of the family.

4- The structure and organization of the family are important factors that significantly affect the behavior of family members.

5- The interactive patterns of the family system strongly shape the behavior of family members.

The conceptual roots of the McMaster model of family functioning were formed more than 50 years ago at McGill University in Montreal, Canada. A team of Epstein-led clinicians and researchers began their work focusing on two major areas of family therapy:

1- Research on non-clinical families

2- Research on the process and outcome of family therapy

A non-clinical family is a family in which none of the members has a psychiatric illness. Such a family may be healthy or unhealthy and have good or poor family functioning.

The model, developed and tested between McGill University and McMaster Hamilton University in Ontario between the mid-1950s and 1970s, was moved to Brown Providence University in Rhode Island, where Epstein moved. And started a family research program, modified and expanded and completed.

Epstein, the founder of family research programs and one of the founders of the model, combined three important models in the field of family therapy to create the final model (McMaster model) and finally inferred the final model. These 3 models were:

1- Individual psychodynamic model

2- Systems model

3- Interactive model.

Individual psychodynamic model

This theory was founded by Adler. Adler was one of Freud's first disciples in the 1920s and founded the Fredergen School of Psychology.

Unlike Freud, who considered instinct to be the main motivation for behavior, and Adel, unlike Yung, who considered primordial forms to be the leader of man, emphasized the social aspect of man.

He also considered the desire for power to be the main source of human energy and motivation, and rejected Freud's "regression" mechanism by not accepting the clear boundary between the conscious and the unconscious.

In Adler's theory, man is a unique, responsible, creative and selective being who has a comprehensive harmony in the dimensions of his personality.

Adler considers man to be inherently a social, creative, and purposeful being whose feelings of inferiority underlie his mental development and always lead him to excellence. In other words, every human being is pushed forward according to this goal. He engages in activities that ultimately determine his or her lifestyle. Therefore, he considers the behavior of the person within his life can be examined. According to Adler, man is the creator of his own destiny and gives meaning to his experiences. According to Adler, abnormal people are not sick, but frustrated people who need hope and courage.

Interactive theory

Interactionist theory considers families as a unit of an interactive personality and tests the symbolic relationship of family members with each other. Within the family, each member is involved with the roles assigned to him or her. Members describe their expectations of their role in each situation of understanding role demands. Members judge their own behavior by examining and interpreting the actions of others in relation to them. The focus of this theory is on the role-playing process. Each role is associated with other roles, and interactions represent a dynamic process for each role. This theory assumes:

- A series of symbols that have a common meaning are obtained during life in a symbolic environment.
- People recognize, evaluate and examine the meaning of symbols.
- Behavior is influenced by the meaning of symbols instead of instincts, needs, commands. Therefore, symbols are important for understanding behavior.
- People learn from culture and become social.
- People's behavior is the result of their life history, which is constantly changing due to new information.

The strength of this theory is the focus on the internal process in families such as roles, conflicts, situations, communication, stress response, decision making and socialization. Therefore, this theory is mostly used by nursing researchers.

The disadvantage of this model is that it is a broad theory and there is no consensus on concepts and assumptions.

Interactionists also consider the family as a relatively closed unit that has less relations with society and the external environment.

The tools used to measure family functioning (McMaster Clinical Rating Scale and McMaster Structured Interview of Family Function) were fully developed in Brown.

In the systems stage in Epstein's work, the family is considered an open system. The structure, organization, and patterns of exchange displayed in the family system were important variables in determining the behavior of family members. Internal or external changes affect the family system and the behavior of all family members. In the treatment of families, disturbance within the system is considered in terms of structure, organization, or exchange patterns. The internal psychological processes of the members of the system are of secondary importance. It is assumed that if the variables of the system work well together, then the behavior of the individual as well as the internal and psychological processes of these individuals are affected.

The McMaster model does not cover all aspects of family functioning but identifies dimensions that are important in the clinical treatment of families. That is, it deals with the current functioning of the family, not with the evolutionary stage of the family or its previous growth. This model divides family responsibilities into three parts. Basic tasks, such as providing food, security, health care for their members, transformational tasks, such as caring for a baby, caring for a family teen, and critical tasks, which include family skills in times of crisis and unexpected events such as a family member's serious illness.

Nurses whose field of work is related to the family and the community to which the family belongs, need special training in assessing the health problems and health needs of the target families, as well as intervening in the planning of health interventions to help families. Therefore, considering that this study was performed on the families of cancer patients and also the field of study of the researcher is community health nursing, in this section, different branches of nursing related to working with families and especially patients' families are described. He has cancer, we will pay.

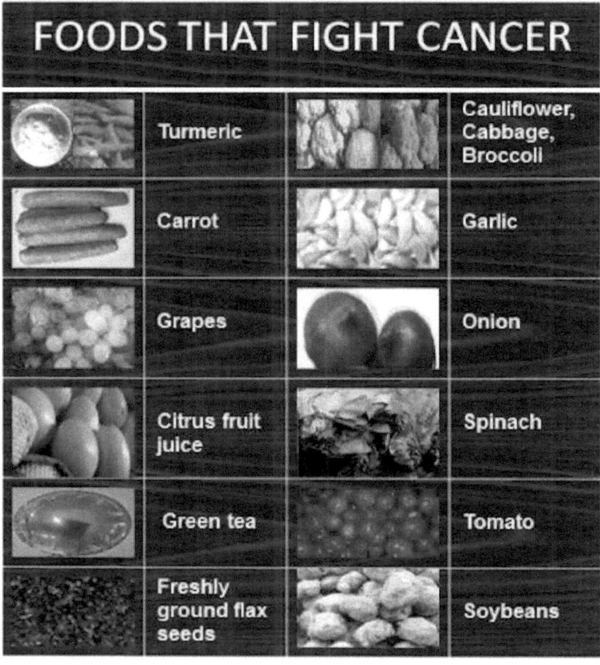

Figure 20. What should eat for cancer patient and what should not

Community Health Nursing

The most important members of the health team are community health nurses. Community health nursing plays a key role in supporting public health and is the act of promoting and protecting public health using the knowledge of nursing, social sciences and community health science. This type of nursing is a systematic process that aims to:

- Assessing and identifying the health needs of communities, families and individuals
- Develop intervention programs to meet health needs
- Evaluation of interventions performed
- Use of process results in health care programs.

Community health nurses are people who work with communities and whose roles focus on primary health, which may involve making community rights decisions without having direct contact with anyone in the community.

Pillars of community health nursing

- Planning for health promotion and health support programs.
- Reducing high-risk behaviors and inequalities in the provision of health services.
- Prevention of diseases.
- Monitoring the health of communities and nations to identify endangered (vulnerable) populations and identify priorities for action.

Family health can affect the health of the community as a whole. The health of communities is measured by the sense of well-being of people and their families. The challenges of a community health nurse are to provide care for communities and nations, not just focus on the level of individuals and families. Families should be considered as part of society. The community health nurse should be aware of the community, and keep in mind that communities are different, not only because of differences in health needs but also because of differences in health resources, to ensure that family and community needs are met, and Consider the different priorities and needs of the family in different communities.

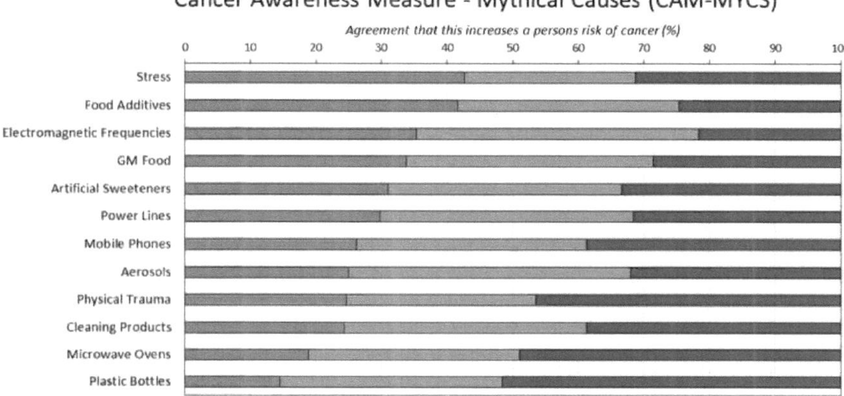

Figure 21. The lifestyle factors that cause cancer

Family Health Nursing

The goal of family health nursing is to help families achieve a higher level of performance in the context of their specific goals, aspirations, and abilities. The practice of family nursing is to provide nursing care to families and their members in various disease / health situations. Family health nursing has a strong theoretical basis and includes nurses and families who interact with each other to enhance the success of the family and its members and disease / health responses.

The family review process is accompanied by ongoing information gathering and professional judgment that is attached to the information gathered. Therefore, an important variable that promotes or prevents family nursing is how the nurse sees the problems. Knowledge and awareness of family theories, as well as the use of a systematic framework for reviewing and working with families, greatly help the nurse to move from individual to family aspects.

Given that the present study is designed in relation to the families of cancer patients, we will have a brief overview of cancer nursing, which is a new branch of nursing.

Cancer nursing is a unique specialty in the nursing profession. In 1986, Ash wrote about cancer nursing, there are always nurses who provide care for a cancer patient, but these nurses do not always have the necessary knowledge and skills. In 1997, Corner listed examples of cancer nursing behavior: being by the patient's side, maintaining patient hope, reducing patient pain, maintaining patient privacy, and anticipating patient needs. Central to the philosophy of cancer nursing is the promotion of self-centered care, believing that patients have the right to be informed about their illness and treatment, and to receive advice on treatment decisions.

The care provided by nurses to families is a vital part of providing care for a person with cancer. Because cancer nurses are in a unique position to provide care and support to cancer survivors and their families during and after diagnosis. These nurses are not only involved in the treatment of the disease, but also have the roles of educator, guide, counselor and advocate for the rights of people with cancer. They also play an important role in promoting patients' health behaviors.

Therefore, the basic dimension in cancer rehabilitation is that the patient and the family are considered as one unit. Nurses, like other members of the medical team, have the opportunity to play an important role in supporting and empowering cancer patients and their families in the course of cancer treatment. Nurses can increase patients' and staff's awareness of cancer rehabilitation needs and develop a positive attitude about cancer rehabilitation by emphasizing that cancer is a chronic disease.

Browse texts

1- In a 2003 study of women with breast cancer in Japan in 2003, the relationship between adaptation responses of cancer patients to breast cancer diagnosis and family functioning was examined. 46 cancer patients and their spouses participated in this study. Patients and their spouses completed the Cancer Mental Judgment Scale (MAC) and the 60-item Family Performance Assessment (FAD) questionnaire without knowing each other's responses and separately.

The MAC itself has 5 dimensions and includes 40 modes that describe how people respond to hearing a cancer diagnosis. This study focuses more on the two dimensions of helplessness / despair and psychological warfare. The patient with a psychological warfare accepts the diagnosis of cancer and searches for information about the cancer and decides to fight it. In contrast, a person with the trait of helplessness / despair is affected by the awareness of cancer diagnosis and their daily life is disrupted.

Patient MAC scale scores from psychological warfare and frustration were entered into the analysis as dependent variables. First, univariate analysis was performed between MAC scale scores.

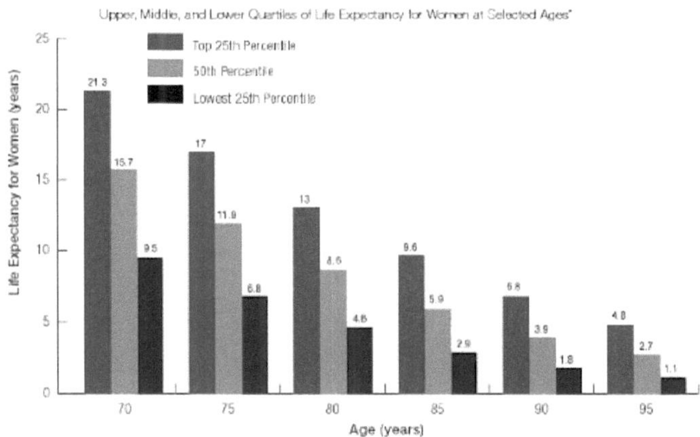

Figure 22. Breast Cancer Survival Rate: Prognosis by Age and More

Psychosocial and biological factors were examined to determine the independent variables with Mann-Whitney, U test or Spearman correlation coefficient.

The results of multiple analyzes showed that patients' perceptions of poor family performance in the FAD scale communication dimension were associated with high MAC scale helplessness / frustration scores. The level of education is inversely related to the psychological warfare dimension on the MAC scale.

The results indicate that there is a relationship between the patient's attitude of helplessness / frustration in dealing with cancer and the communication dimension in the family. Therefore, in addition to the patient, the staff of the health team should pay attention to other family members and try to promote good communication patterns among family members.

- Another study entitled "Family Function and Stress in Breast Cancer Patients and Families" was conducted in 2005 with the aim of gaining a view of family functioning in breast cancer patients and their families. Criteria for inclusion in the study, diagnosis at any stage of breast cancer, knowledge of cancer diagnosis, age over 20 years, 3 months after diagnosis, sufficient physical strength to answer questions, no cognitive impairment and concomitant malignancy All samples completed 3 scales: FRI (Family Relationship Index), SAS (Zong Anxiety Scale) and SDS (Zong Depression Scale). 3 types of family structure scale were classified into 3 clusters Cluster 1 was called supportive family structure which such families showed a low level of psychological stress among their members Cluster 2 Medium family structure, which these families They have moderate cohesion and clarity of communication and low conflict. Cluster of 3 families with conflict, whose tensions are constantly Appropriate communication is involved during treatment.

After this division, individuals' perceptions of family functioning were compared in 3 categories and the psychological stress of family members was analyzed using SDS and SAS scales using ANOVA test. Cluster analysis yielded 3 groups of patients and their families. One type with high coherence, high resolution and low conflict (46. (n = type with supporting conflict, low coherence, high resolution and high conflict) (n=60) medium type with limited coherence, limited resolution and low conflict) (n=60)

The findings of this study showed that family performance typology can psychologically identify at-risk families. A family-centered approach can help reduce stress, especially in families with conflict. Therefore, medical team staff should focus on other family members in addition to the patient and intervene to promote good communication patterns in family members, because the supportive family structure leads to a sense of family well-being.

Another study was conducted in 2007 by Mantani at the University of Hiroshima, Japan, entitled "Factors Related to Anxiety and Depression in Women with Breast

Cancer and Their Husbands: The Role of Insensitivity and Family Function." The aim of this study was to investigate insensitivity, family functioning and other factors that may affect the level of anxiety and depression in women with breast cancer and their husbands. In this cross-sectional study, 46 women with breast cancer who underwent surgery and their husbands were studied.

All samples completed 3 scales: FAD (Family Function Assessment Tool), SAS (Zong Anxiety Scale) and SDS (Zong Depression Scale). Participants also completed the TAS-20 Scale, which measures 20 items of insensitivity. The Japanese version of FAD has 60 items and has been used to examine 7 dimensions of family performance. A higher score indicates poorer family performance. For statistical analysis, a univariate analysis between SDS and SAS was performed first, and socio-demographic, psychological, and medical factors were used to determine independent variables by Mann-Whitney test or Spearman correlation coefficient in patients and Spouses were assessed. Then, the final risk factors of SAS and SDS of patients were determined as dependent variables using multiple regression analysis with their spouses' scores. The findings showed that family functioning is associated with depression in cancer patients and their spouses, but Family-related performance of depression varies among patients and their husbands.

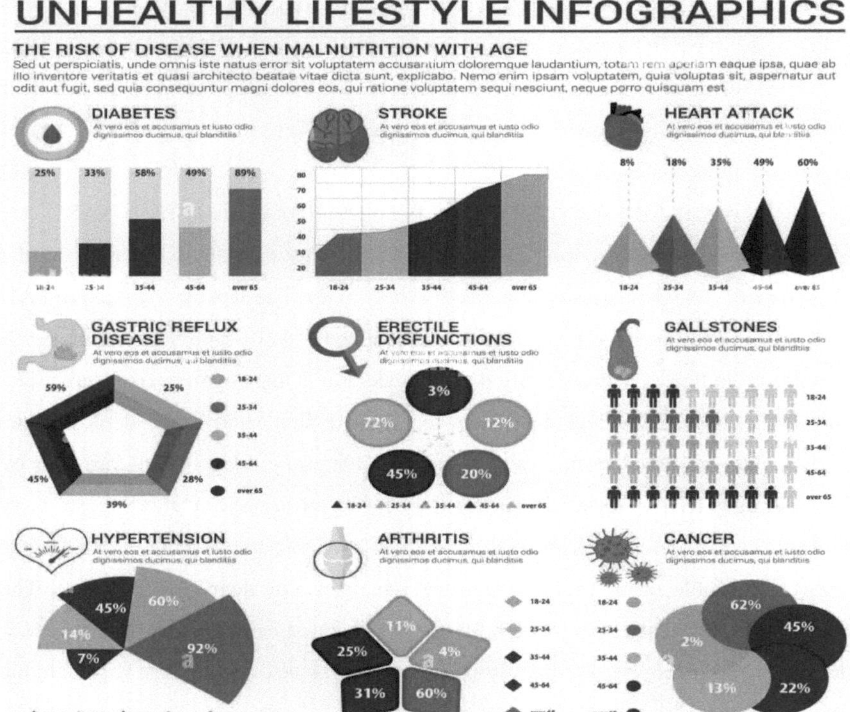

Figure 23. Unhealthy lifestyle infographics. Graph, chart and diagram shows the risk of diabetes, cancer,

Patients' depression is related to their perception of inappropriate emotional response among family members. While husbands' perception of inappropriate roles in family members is related to their depression. In other words, if the patient is unable to receive an empathetic response from the family during times of stress, the patient's depression becomes more severe. Possible links between family relationships, children's performance with parents with cancer, and family environment. The study was conducted over a 2-year period at the Medical University of Croningen. Inclusion criteria were 1 to 5 years after the diagnosis of cancer, having a child aged 4-18 years and fluency in Dutch. The study focused on 209 families and focused on families with children between the ages of 11 and 18. In total, 138 patients, 114 patients' spouses and 221 children completed the environmental questionnaire. Patients and their families completed the CBCL Children Behavior Checklist and adolescents completed the YSR Children Self-Reporting Questionnaire.

T-test was used to compare family members 'reports of family environment and patients' reports of family performance with reports of parents, spouses with adolescents and differences between reports of girls and boys.

Pearson correlation coefficient was used to explain the relationship between adolescents' performance and their reports of cancer-related stress, as well as each family member's perception of the family environment and parent-adolescent differences. Correlation coefficient less than 0.30 was considered as weak, 0.30-0.50 as moderate and more than 0.50 as strong. Compared to the normal group, parents organized their families with less conflict. They found better and less control and more social than the norm group.

The FRI, or family relationship index, was significantly higher than the norm group, and the FSI, or family structure index, was similar to the norm group.

No significant differences were found between patients 'and spouses' reports of family performance. Adolescents also reported that their families were more cohesive, more social, better organized, and less conflicted than normal groups.

The findings of this study indicate that families with one parent with cancer (both adolescents and the parents themselves) are more positive.

In 2008, Schmitt conducted a study on cancer patients and their children with the aim of testing family-related factors in such patients. The hypothesis of this study was that "the presence of cancer in one parent could be one.

Explaining the cause of the relationship between the presence of chronic disease in the family and family functioning in terms of problem solving, we can say that the existence of the disease and its persistence in families, causes families to change their functional areas. In these families, the strategies used to deal with and control the disease are often ineffective or not done properly. Therefore, according to the results of the present study, it can be concluded that Iranian families' strategies for coping with the disease are probably more efficient and effective, and both patients and their spouses are involved in issues that occur in the family due to cancer. They are not. This may be due to the fact that cancer patients face many problems and need to strengthen their problem-solving skills over time, so that they do not have problems after family functioning and on the other hand again given that the more positive interaction between couples, the more problem-solving skills occur, the more the couple's negative interaction increases, the less problem-solving or negotiation skills occur. The reason for the difference in the findings could probably be the existence of positive interactions in families and among Iranian couples.

According to Clark, problem solving and communication are considered as the most important dimensions of family functioning. The results of the study conducted by Smith on cancer patients and their children to determine family functioning indicate that according to the children and parents participating in the study, family functioning, in general, is appropriate and communication in these families is disrupted.

In another multicenter study in several European countries to determine family functioning and its relationship to emotional and behavioral problems of adolescents with cancer parents, adolescents in the study, when one parent has cancer, Family performance in communication and other dimensions have been better reported. The results of studies conducted in other countries show that families with a person with cancer or other chronic diseases such as mental illness, chronic gastrointestinal problems and epilepsy, have weakened communication. Also, in the study of interfering factors in patients' judgments about breast cancer, it was observed that there is a communication disorder that is associated with frustration in women. It seems that this discrepancy can be due to differences in the nature, type and specific physical and psychological effects in different diseases.

The communication dimension is the only variable of family functioning that has a significant relationship with patients' anxiety and patients with communication disorders experience higher levels of anxiety. Therefore, it can be reported that patients participating in the present study may have experienced less anxiety.

Establishing healthy and empathetic communication patterns between couples, one of whom has cancer, helps them to have a positive and realistic assessment of stress and a mutual understanding of cancer and its effects, as well as important issues. Reach their own lives. The results of the present study can indicate that the couples participating in this study were able to establish healthy communication patterns in the family and were able to have a positive assessment of stress in the event of a family crisis and to adapt to it effectively.

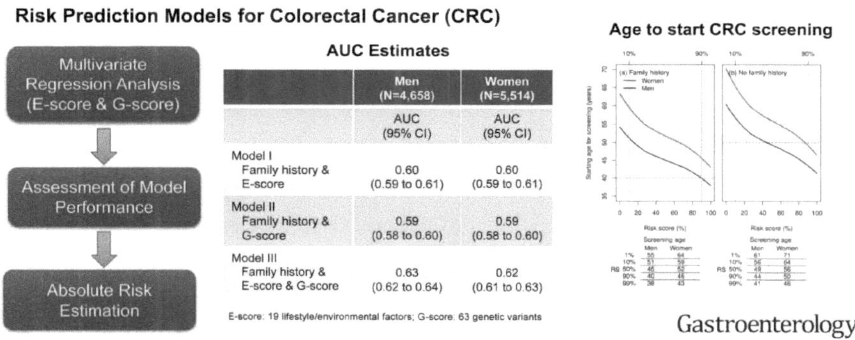

	Men (N=4,658)	Women (N=5,514)
	AUC (95% CI)	AUC (95% CI)
Model I Family history & E-score	0.60 (0.59 to 0.61)	0.60 (0.59 to 0.61)
Model II Family history & G-score	0.59 (0.58 to 0.60)	0.59 (0.58 to 0.60)
Model III Family history & E-score & G-score	0.63 (0.62 to 0.64)	0.62 (0.61 to 0.63)

Figure 24. Determining Risk of Colorectal Cancer and Starting Age of Screening Based on Lifestyle

The results of the present study in line with the third goal of the study entitled "Study of family function in the dimension of roles when cancer occurs in one of the couples" showed that in the eyes of patients and their healthy spouses, family function in the dimension of roles is not disturbed and within normal limits. There is also no statistically significant difference between the scores obtained by cancer patients in terms of roles and the scores obtained by their healthy spouses in this area. In other words, it seems that the roles in the studied families have not been affected by cancer. The results of a study conducted in European countries on cancer patients and their children showed that the perception of children and parents about family functioning was positive and then the roles in these families were not impaired. In 2007, a study was conducted in the Netherlands to examine the relationship between family functioning and the emotional and behavioral problems of adolescents with cancer parents. Participants in the study were couples, one of whom had cancer and met the inclusion criteria. The results showed that family functioning has improved in terms of communication and other dimensions of family functioning. The family is not disturbed in the role dimension.

However, according to Given, there is evidence that in the advanced stages of the disease, changes in the roles of family members occur and the burden imposed on caregivers reduces the quality of life of patients and their families. Also, the wives of women with breast cancer, in addition to playing their roles, also take on the roles of their husbands. Children of parents with cancer, in turn, experience a change in role, especially when their mothers are ill. Take care of the house. Therefore, when the results of the present study show that the dimension of family roles is not affected by cancer, it seems that the lack of change in roles in these families on the one hand indicates a positive and decisive effect of culture. On the other hand, it indicates the existence of special family relations in crisis situations among Iranian families. Because the impact of diagnosing a threatening disease such as cancer on the functioning of families depends greatly on the culture and social relations that govern society. As a result, it is not easy to generalize the findings of different societies about the family and its components.

The results of the present study in line with the fourth goal of the study entitled "Evaluation of family performance in the dimension of emotional response during cancer in one of the couples" showed that patients and their spouses function in the dimension of emotional response is not impaired and is within normal limits. Also, there is no statistically significant difference between the scores obtained by cancer patients in terms of emotional response and the scores obtained by their healthy spouses in this area. In some studies, conducted in different countries to determine the performance of patients' families and their children, the results showed that the performance of families in cancer patients and their children was not impaired in terms of emotional response.

Also, in a study conducted in the Netherlands, to examine the relationship between family functioning and emotional and behavioral problems of adolescents with parents with cancer, it was found that from the point of view of children and parents, family performance has improved in terms of emotional response. Chronic diseases have also been impaired in the dimension of emotional responsiveness of family functioning. For example, when examining the family performance of parents who have undergone brain surgery, there is a disturbance in the emotional response dimension in their children's reports, or when examining the family performance of patients with epilepsy, there is a disturbance in this dimension.

Also, men with chronic depression have impaired emotional responsiveness that is significantly associated with the severity of their depression. However, in the families studied in the present study, the emotional responsiveness of the family is quantitatively and qualitatively proportional to the stressful situation. In justifying the contradictions in the findings of the present study and reviewing the literature, it can be said that how family members respond to stress can affect the mental state of patients. In other words, when the patient cannot receive an empathetic response from the family during times of stress, the patient's depression intensifies. In confirmation of this, the Fiber study in 2011 also showed that sick men have higher scores in terms of emotional responsiveness than sick women, and as a result, their severity of depression is higher. In such families, the ability to express emotions, both positive and negative, is impaired. Impaired intimacy and closeness between family members may be one of the reasons for families' poor performance in terms of emotional responsiveness. Therefore, in the studied families, the intimacy between the couples probably prevented the disruption in this dimension.

However, in the studied families, where the emotional response dimension is not disturbed, families are probably able to express their emotions, which is due to the existence of intimacy in the families. The results of the present study are in line with the fifth goal of the study entitled "When cancer occurs in one of the couples" showed that in the eyes of patients and their healthy spouses, the family function in the dimension of emotional intercourse is not disturbed and is within the normal range, and also among the scores obtained by cancer patients in the dimension of emotional intercourse And there are no statistically significant differences in the scores obtained by their healthy spouses in this area.

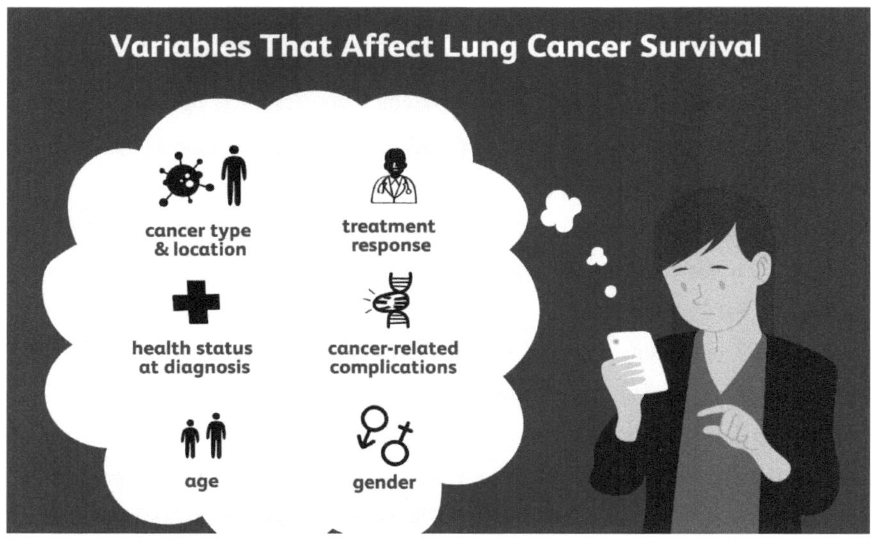

Figure 25. What Is Stage 2 Lung Cancer Life Expectancy?

The results of Mellis' research showed that families with organs with cancer have disorders in the dimension of emotional intercourse (Mellis 2009). Sochini also confirmed in his study that improper performance in the dimension of emotional intercourse is directly related to the degree of frustration in patients.

In a study conducted on families with a parent with cancer, after emotional intercourse in their children's reports, the family function was not disrupted and is in the normal range. The findings of this group of studies are consistent with the present study. Some studies have even reported an improvement in the emotional dimension of family functioning after a member has cancer. These three types of findings, namely, improved family functioning in terms of emotional intercourse, worsening performance, and being in the normal range, may be due to the fact that couples in different societies use different methods of communication. Because family psychologists acknowledge that proper communication increases couples' emotional intimacy. If couples can communicate in the right ways, not only will they have effective communication with each other, but their intimacy will also increase. On the other hand, increasing the intimacy and emotional companionship of the couple, increases their sensitivity to each other, thus increasing their emotional intercourse. Therefore, considering that the dimension of communication in the families studied in this study is in the normal range, consequently the dimension of emotional intercourse has also been reported in the normal range. These findings can confirm that the couples studied were able to understand each other to a large extent and were able to have an effective and correct understanding of each other's interests and needs.

The results of the present study in line with the sixth goal of the study entitled "Study of family performance dimension in behavior control dimension when cancer occurs in one of the couples" showed that in the eyes of patients and their healthy spouses, family function in behavior control dimension is not disturbed and within normal limits. There is also no statistically significant difference between the scores obtained by cancer patients in terms of behavior control and the scores obtained by their healthy spouses in this area. They use unhealthy patterns of behavior control and the other half of the families do not have a disorder in the dimension of behavior control. Also, in reviewing the texts done in different societies and cultures, when cancer or other chronic diseases occur, the dimension of controlling family behavior is reported to be appropriate and within the normal range. Consistent with the results of the present study. Therefore, it can be concluded that the families participating in this study and other studies mentioned that have chronic patients, among the four methods of behavior control, have used the method of rational authority (which is the best type of behavior control than dry methods). Or disturbed and inefficient. In reviewing the literature, some studies on the families of cancer patients have reported the overall performance of the family in line with the present study and in the normal range and some even better than Normal range has been reported, and general functional dysfunction has also occurred in families with organs with other chronic diseases.

Some studies have also shown that having one parent with cancer impairs the overall functioning of the family, especially when the man in the family becomes ill. Disorders in the overall functioning of the family have a significant positive relationship with the mental and psychological conditions of family children.

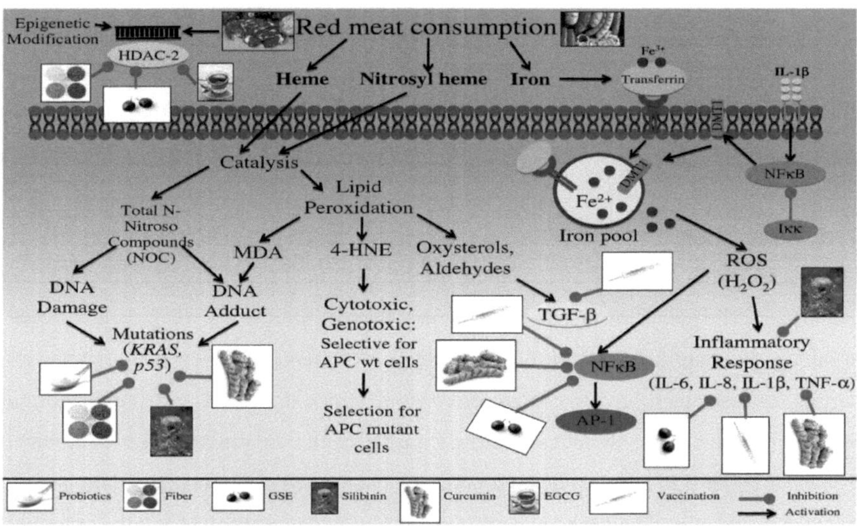

Figure 26. Identifying Molecular Targets of Lifestyle Modifications in Colon Cancer Prevention

In this dimension of family performance, when reviewing texts, we are again faced with 3 types of results. Results consistent with the present study that reported overall family functioning within the normal range, studies that reported overall performance above the normal range, and studies that reported overall overall family functioning as poor. The reason for the discrepancy in the findings may be that when experiencing an illness or crisis, the family, if able to strengthen family ties and act as a whole, can withstand the emotional transformation that follows the illness. Since the emotional relationships between Iranian families have deep roots, it prevents the family from wavering during a crisis. Researchers have proven that there is a statistically significant relationship between the duration of marriage and marital satisfaction, probably because of this relationship. It could be that as the duration of marriage increases, couples become more aware of each other's emotions and can better understand each other.

Also, employed, housewife and self-employed patients performed better than retired or university-employed patients. In other cases, there was no statistically significant relationship between overall family functioning and some characteristics of spouses of cancer patients.

Findings show that there is a relationship between education level and quality of life of cancer patients. Also, there is no significant relationship between gender, age, occupation and social status and quality of life of patients. However, there is a relationship between the number of chemotherapy courses in cancer patients and quality of life. The mentioned studies have compared the relationship of some demographic characteristics of cancer patients with their quality of life and not with family performance. However, some studies in other countries have not reported a significant relationship between participants' demographic characteristics and overall family performance score.

According to the literature mentioned above, the results of the analysis of the presence or absence of a relationship between family performance and demographic characteristics of participants, in some demographic characteristics show consistency with previous studies, but in some characteristics, there is a discrepancy. The reason for this discrepancy in studies can be related to differences in the level of social welfare and the ceiling of support of different organizations such as insurers in different countries, especially developing countries. Even among the patients participating in this study, there was a difference in the level of support from insurance companies and other organizations to which patients were affiliated. Therefore, given these differences, one cannot expect common results on the relationship between patients' demographics and family functioning.

Chapter III

Lung Cancer

Cancer is a genetic disease that results from the uncontrolled growth and division of cells in a part of the body that results from the effects of environmental factors and genetic disorders. In other words, cancer occurs as a result of a series of mutations in human genes. There are more than 200 types of cancer today, one of the most common of which is lung cancer.

Lung cancer is the second most common cancer among men and women and is one of the most preventable cancers. There are generally two types of lung cancer:

1) Small cell lung cancer (SCLC)

2) Non-small cell lung cancer (NSCLC)

How they both grow and spread in the body and how they are treated is different. Lung cancers are classified under the microscope based on the appearance of the cells. Non-small cell lung cancer (NSCLC) is also divided into three categories: 1) superficial tissue cancer, 2) mucosal and lymph node carcinoma (glandular epithelium), and 3) large cell lung cancer. Among people with this type of cancer, about 90-85% of cases are NSCLC and about 10-15% of cases are SCLC.

The most common clinical symptoms of lung cancer include persistent and chronic cough, chest pain, anorexia, weight loss, sputum, shortness of breath, respiratory infections such as bronchitis, the onset of wheezing, etc., which usually do not appear in the early stages of the disease. Therefore, the mortality rate of this type of cancer is very high.

Health has been around since the creation of man for many centuries, but wherever it is mentioned, its physical dimension has been considered and less attention has been paid to its mental and social dimensions. Health means ability to adapt, effective communication, responsibility, good nutrition, good physical function, stress management, good mood and effective social functioning. The World Health Organization considers "health to be a condition of physical, mental and social well-being and not merely a cure for disease".

The main challenge of health in the twentieth century is survival and the challenge of the present century is a better quality of life. Nowadays, in addition to calculating mortality, frequency and severity of disease, health diagnosis and evaluation of health interventions pay attention to other human values such as quality of life. Quality of life is a broader concept of health that encompasses a range of physical, mental and social well-being. In fact, quality of life has a multidimensional structure that is examined in various functional, social, psychological and emotional dimensions.

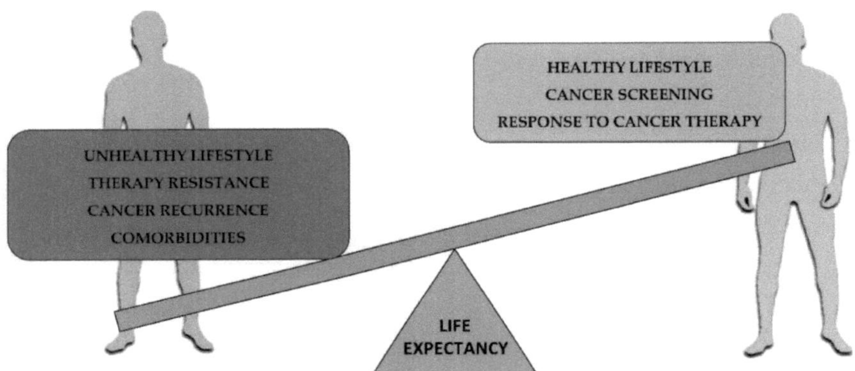

Figure 27. Micro RNAs Patterns as Potential Tools for Diagnostic and Prognostic Follow

There is a correlation between disease and quality of life and physical disorders related to disease have a direct effect on all aspects of quality of life. Chronic diseases are among the disorders that severely affect people's health and consequently their quality of life. Chronic illness is a condition that disrupts daily activities for more than 3 months a year or causes hospitalization for more than one month a year or at the time of diagnosis. The development of technology and drug treatment has increased the number of children suffering from chronic diseases.

Approximately 10-40% of children in the world suffer from chronic diseases. The impact of chronic and debilitating diseases on the performance and health status of the child is very high. These children need to rest in bed 3 times more than other children, and 2 times more than other children need a doctor, and 5 times more are hospitalized. Chronic illness can last for years or last a lifetime and affects all activities of children and parents. Among chronic diseases, cancer is one of the cases that has always been on the human mind.

Cancer is a general term for complex diseases that result from certain genetic changes that cause uncontrolled and irregular cell proliferation. The term pediatric cancer refers to cases of cancer that are diagnosed in children under 15 years of age. Pediatric cancer consists of a group of malignancies, each of which has different epidemiological characteristics, biological characteristics, treatment methods, and survival problems. Cancer creates unfavorable physical, psychological, social and economic conditions for the family and society and causes many years of the patient's life to be spent dealing with the disease and pursuing treatment methods.

As the incidence of childhood diseases (especially infectious diseases) has decreased in industrialized and developing countries, the number of children diagnosed with cancer has increased. In Europe and the United States, the disease is reported to be the leading cause of death in children aged 5-14 years and its prevalence in this age group is approximately 129 per million.

A study conducted by Mahak (Institute for the Protection of Children with Cancer) on the prevalence of cancer in Iran shows that during different years in the country, the number of children with cancer was 9 out of every 100,000 children per year. The number increased to 15 children in 2008. According to the report of Fars Province Cancer Registration Center, from 2001 to 2008 (for 8 years), the number of children with cancer was 1610, among which blood cancers were the most common (47.8%), followed by tumors. The brain and other parts of the central nervous system (9.5%) and lymph nodes (9.3%) have the most cases.

Today, with the development of medical science and related technology, cancer in children and adolescents has gradually changed from an acute and fatal disease to a chronic disease and the survival rate has increased. Currently, more than 50% of children suffering from cancer survive about 5 years or more and reach adulthood. Despite the increase in survival, cancer provides life-threatening conditions and causes fundamental changes in the child and family.

On the other hand, the increase in aggressive therapies causes children to experience unpleasant physical, mental and behavioral complications during treatment, and this raises many questions about the quality of life of children during survival. Lack of control of these complications intensifies the negative effects on the quality of life of these patients and may neutralize any advantage of this increase in survival due to the increased cost of side effects.

The quality of life of the sick child, as a result of the pain caused by the disease itself and aggressive treatment methods, as well as reduced energy to enjoy normal daily activities, inability to communicate with friends at school and community, and fear of the future, are endangered. Therapies cause the child to be constantly tired and sick.

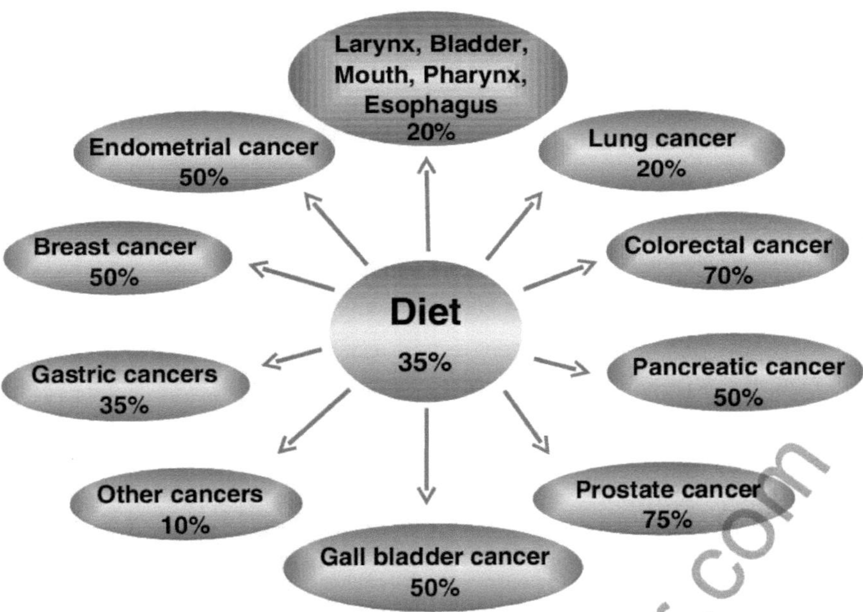

Figure 28. Cancer is a Preventable Disease that Requires Major Lifestyle Changes

These children are also prone to infection and are constantly hospitalized, leading to the child being separated from family, school and community. Cancer treatments are associated with complications and toxicity that endanger the quality of life in the short or long term. Therapies such as chemotherapy, radiation therapy or surgery may have adverse effects on childhood development and cause long-term physical, psychological and social effects in childhood and adulthood.

All of these events trigger psychological reactions such as depression, anxiety, low self-esteem, and impaired mental image of the child. Feelings of depression in children with cancer affect the quality of life and the ability to treat. The results of William Lee et al. Showed that more than half of children with cancer were at risk for depression and suicidal ideation and needed special attention by health care providers. Restriction of social and family activities disrupts the child's natural development, activities, and social interactions over a long period of time. Medical expenses, length of hospital stay and psychological problems caused by this disease indicate the weight of the socio-economic burden arising from it.

Research has shown that the presence of a chronic disease such as cancer can affect the patient's quality of life in various dimensions and impair his quality of life. The results of the findings of Yaris et al. In Turkey showed that all aspects of the quality of life of these children have been significantly impaired. This has made the quality of life the focus of treatments offered to children with cancer. The goal of the treatments used today for children with cancer is not only to increase survival but also to increase the quality of life of these children. Although survival and health status are relatively easy to assess, they often do not reflect the full effect of cancer and treatment on the child. Such treatment and disease outcomes are achieved by assessing health-related quality of life.

Health-related quality of life can be considered as an operational tool for measuring overall health and well-being and is now referred to as a key indicator that should be routinely considered in health research. Quality of life is a comprehensive concept that encompasses all physical, psychological, cognitive, social, cultural and economic dimensions of one's life. In the physical dimension, the most important aspect is the state of a person's performance. Perception of quality of life is affected by a person's ability at different ages to continue to function and perform daily activities such as taking care of themselves, going to school and the workplace. In the psychological dimension, it should be said that mental health is an important component of quality of life and having a positive attitude is effective in improving the quality of life. In the socio-cultural dimension, the roles of each individual in the family and society and his social relationships are factors affecting the quality of life.

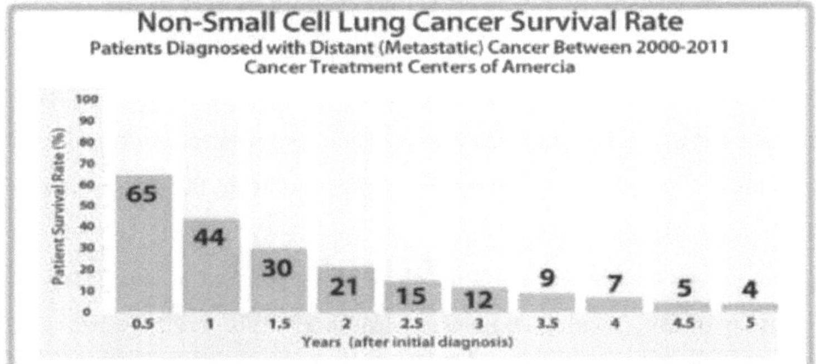

Figure 29. lung cancer

The specific quality of life of children with cancer shows the impact of disease and treatment as well as the effects of treatment on a person's quality of life. Quality of life in children with cancer is a general sense of well-being based on the ability to participate in routine activities, interact with others, and adapt to distressing cognitive, emotional, and physical events, and to create a sense of illness experience. Quality of life assessment is an important aspect in the treatment of children with cancer and is a way that allows the child to express their fears and concerns during the treatment process. Because the quality-of-life assessment information quantitatively demonstrates the effect of treatment on a child's performance, it is a very valuable criterion for sick children, families, and treatment teams to decide on the benefits and costs of different treatments for pediatric cancers. This knowledge can be used to identify a group of children who are expected to have a low quality of life, to use care and supportive interventions to improve their health and also to improve the relationship between the patient and the treatment team. Increases patient and family satisfaction with the treatment team.

Measuring the quality of life in cancer patients is expanding rapidly. Although patients' perceptions of quality of life are an important element in assessing health-related quality of life, parents or Child caregivers are used. Having children with a chronic illness can cause psychological stress to parents and reduce their ability to cope with events. Diagnosis and treatment of cancer creates psychological stress that often has a negative effect on parents' mental health. Psychological reactions such as anxiety, depression, denial, anger, and loss of self-confidence are observed in parents due to fear of recurrence of the disease and the future of the child. In addition, the financial and physical problems of treatment expose parents to a great deal of stress, which harms their general health. Decreased parental health affects the quality of life of their children and makes parents feel that their child's health is very vulnerable, resulting in excessive protection and limitation of the child by parents and adverse effects on the child. On the contrary, better parental adjustment improves the child's quality of life and the child will be better able to adapt to the stressors imposed by the disease. The results of Oriental et al.'s study showed that child disease is associated with maternal depression in case of blood malignancies (p <0.001) and in case of thalassemia (p <0.015). Provide the necessary psychological support for the child and parents to adapt to illness and treatment.

Most quality-of-life studies have been performed on children with cancer, and a limited number of studies have identified factors affecting the quality of life of children with cancer during treatment. Different dimensions of quality of life such as cognitive, emotional, physical is changed by individual-social and psychological-social variables. Research on chronic diseases has shown that health-related quality of life varies according to individual-social characteristics such as income level, educational status, employment status, and people who do not have desirable individual-social characteristics have a lower quality of life.

These associations have been reported in a wide range of diseases such as cancer, AIDS, lupus, kidney disease, and mental disorders, and an inverse relationship between quality of life related to child health and individual socio-variables such as low parental education, low family income that causes stress. Psychology of parents and family members becomes there. Other risk factors associated with low quality of life in children and adolescents with cancer are limited resources and increased family stressors and the number of family members. Social support is recognized as the strongest force for coping successfully and easily with people in the face of cancer and stressful situations. Cancer patients who receive social support have a higher quality of life. There is also a significant relationship between socio-economic status and quality of life. The better the economic, social, psychological, psychological and family status of cancer patients, the higher their quality of life.

A number of studies have shown that the age at which cancer is diagnosed is a factor that affects children's performance. Children who develop cancer at an early age suffer more from their educational and psychological functioning. These children suffer from psychological problems in the two areas of social adjustment with peers and emotional health. Other studies have refuted this hypothesis. But the findings show that children with cancer have more emotional and social problems than their healthy peers.

The results of Zelzero et al.'s research showed that female gender, income below $ 20,000 and lack of health insurance are associated with poor quality of life. Musk et al. Also identified factors associated with low quality of life in children with cancer and found that there was a significant relationship between fatigue ($p < 0.02$) and delayed complications ($p < 0.01$) with low physical function, fatigue ($p < 0.0001$). There is a low social class ($p < 0.04$) and a diagnosis of brain tumor ($p < 0.01$) with low psychological function.

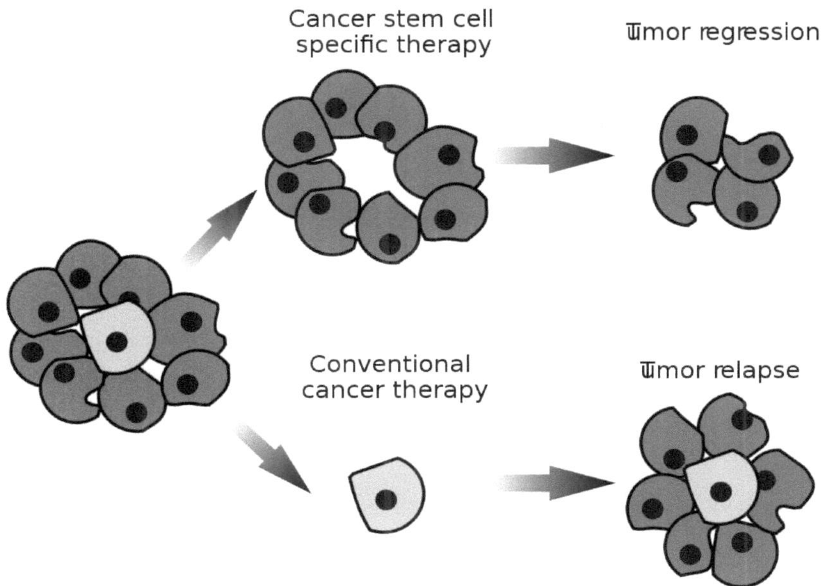

Figure 30. Cancer stem cell

In another study by Sang et al., older children (p <0.003), girls compared to boys (p <0.007), low-income patients (p <0.01), and being a single parent (P <0.006) was associated with low quality of life. While in another study conducted by Sitarsimi, no statistically significant relationship was found between gender, child birth rank in the family, socio-economic status, parents' education level and health-related quality of life. The results of Barakat et al.'s findings also showed that individual-social variables (sex, age of the child, age of parents) and clinical variables (type of cancer, time of diagnosis and type of treatment) had no significant relationship with quality of life. The results of Forlang's findings in the United States also confirm this.

Characteristics of cancer and its treatment include: type of cancer, type and severity of treatment are related to the quality of life of children and adolescents. The course of treatment, the methods used for treatment, and the side effects are determined by the type and stage of the malignancy, all of which affect the quality of life of the child.

Landolt et al. Showed that quality of life decreases during the childhood cancer treatment process, while most aspects of quality of life improve after treatment. Regardless of the stage of treatment, quality of life has a lot to do with the severity of treatment and the presence of side effects.

Spechley et al. Note that quality of life is associated with the type of cancer and its treatment. In fact, the quality of life in children with cancer is different from different types of cancer, and these differences can help to identify more vulnerable children and their needs and intervention to improve the quality of life. Studies have shown that children with brain tumors experience a more severe illness and treatment period than other types of cancer, especially children with a diagnosis of acute lymphoblastic leukemia. In general, among childhood cancers, children with solid cancers experience adverse effects for a longer period of time, because combined therapies such as surgery, chemotherapy, and radiation therapy are used to treat these cancers.

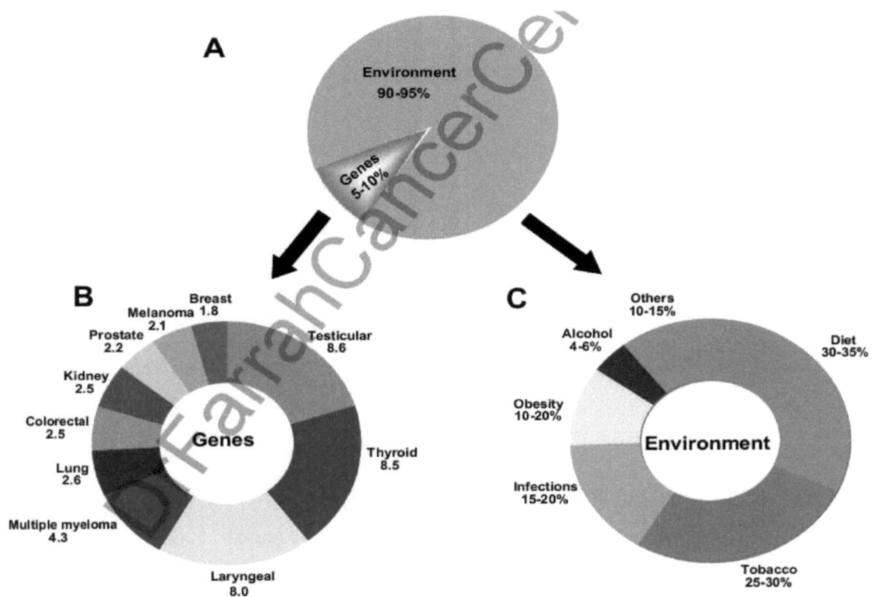

Figure 31. Shree Damodar College of Commerce & Economics

As a result, the quality of life of these children is lower than that of children with leukemia. In addition, the intensity of treatment is an important issue for patients and families of children with cancer, so that severe treatment courses disrupt the functioning of the child and family and may have adverse effects on quality of life.

The type of treatment used to treat children with cancer can affect a child's quality of life both during and after treatment. Studies have shown that children who undergo surgery have a better quality of life than radiotherapy and chemotherapy. Also, chemotherapy is associated with several complications such as fatigue, nausea, vomiting, anemia and alopecia, etc., which can negatively affect the quality of life. Sang et al. Also identified children with cancer with low quality of life and found that children with leukemia had a better quality of life (p <0.0001) in the physical dimension, while more severe treatments (p <0.0002) had a better quality of life. Were lower in association. The results of Begol et al.'s study also showed that children with brain tumors had lower quality of life in social, emotional, physical and educational areas than children with Hodgkin's and non-Hodgkin's lymphoma (001). (P <0.001) and children who received radiation therapy had lower educational performance than children who did not receive radiation (p <0.001).

Given the prevalence of cancer and the importance of its impact on all aspects of life of patients and less attention of our society to the concept of quality of life and related factors, recognizing these factors helps health workers to improve their activities Organize health and improve quality of life. Nurses have a key role in promoting care outcomes among the health care team and improving the quality of life is one of the important responsibilities of nurses. Because nurses have a close relationship with these patients, they can examine the impact of cancer and its characteristics on quality of life and identify the physical, emotional, and psychological needs of these children. In fact, helping nursing children with cancer during treatment to relieve the psychological burden of cancer is the primary responsibility of nurses. Proper nursing interventions reduce the emotional problems and anxiety of these children during the treatment process in the hospital and also reduce the side effects of treatment and improve their quality of life. This group of medical team can help the family to cope with problems and adapt to the disease and provide the necessary support for the family.

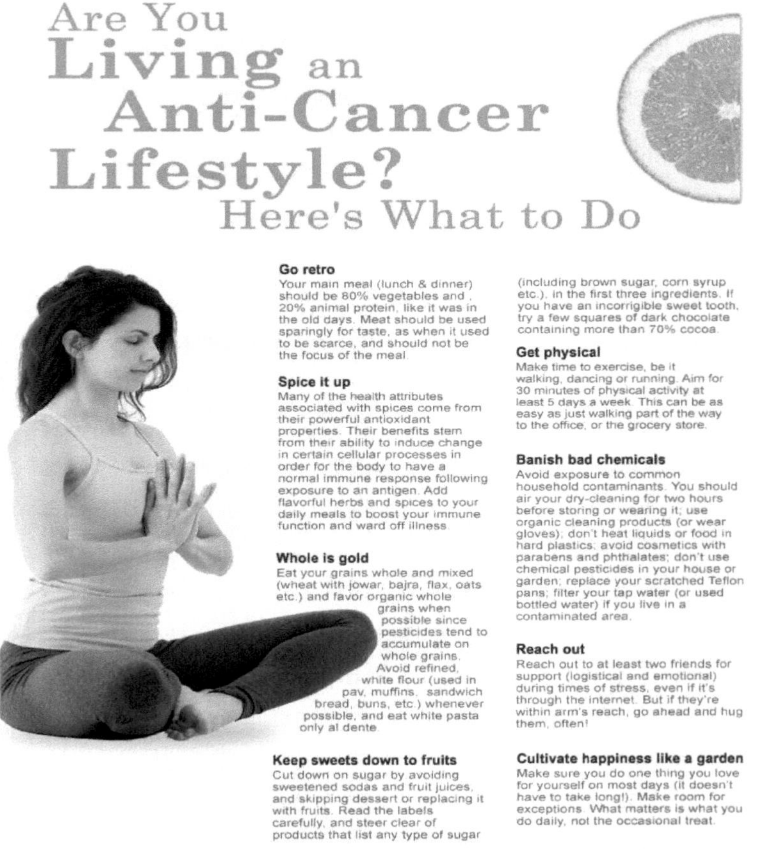

Figure 32. Are you living an anti-cancer lifestyle?

Quality of life is affected by many factors such as culture, age of diagnosis, prognosis, types of medical treatment and predisposing factors that nurses cannot control and influence. But there are factors such as: environmental factors, social and personal status, symptom control that nurse can improve the quality of life of these people by giving the necessary information to the patient and family members and controlling symptoms and complications. Compared to a wide range of cancer studies, there are few research studies on the quality of life of children with cancer. Considering that planning to improve the health of patients requires sufficient information about different aspects of the quality of life of these patients, the researcher decided to conduct a study to investigate the factors related to the quality of life of children with cancer, to Through it, to realize the dimensions of quality of life that are mostly affected by the disease and individual-social factors and factors related to the disease, and need more attention and planning. It is hoped that this research will take a step towards addressing the factors that improve the quality of life of children with cancer.

Chapter IV

Definition of Words

1) Cancer

Theoretical definition: Cancer is a combination of diseases, which occurs due to various changes in genes and causes uncontrolled and irregular cell proliferation that can occur anywhere in the body.

2) A child with cancer

Practical definition: In this study, children with cancer are children aged 2-14 years in whom the diagnosis of cancer has been confirmed by an oncologist and for treatment and follow-up have referred to the oncology department of Amir Hospital and Imam Reza Clinic in Shiraz.

3) Health-related quality of life

Theoretical definition: The World Health Organization means quality of life in the sense of understanding and perception of each individual from his position in life according to the cultural conditions and value system, the society in which he lives and this understanding in relation to the main goals, perceptions and The individual's perceptions of life are meaningful. This fact has a wide range that is influenced in various ways by the individual's physical, mental, personal beliefs and social relationships.

Practical definition: In this study, we mean the total points that are obtained from the answers of the mothers of the studied units to the questions of the health-related quality of life questionnaire. This questionnaire in the age group of 2_5 years (TAPQOL) includes 6 dimensions of physical function: sleep (four cases), appetite (three cases), lung (three cases), stomach (three cases) and skin (three cases), motor function: activity Motor skills (four cases), social functioning: communication (three cases) and behavioral issues (seven cases), cognitive function: cognitive problems (four cases), negative moods: anxiety (three cases), positive moods: positive mood (Three cases) and vitality (three cases) and in the age group of 6_14 years (TACQOL) include seven physical dimensions, automatic activities, social activities, cognitive activities, motor activities, positive moods and negative moods. Each dimension contains eight questions. The scoring of this questionnaire is 5 points in Likert method and scores higher than the average are a sign of good quality of life. (Discussed in detail in the data collection tool).

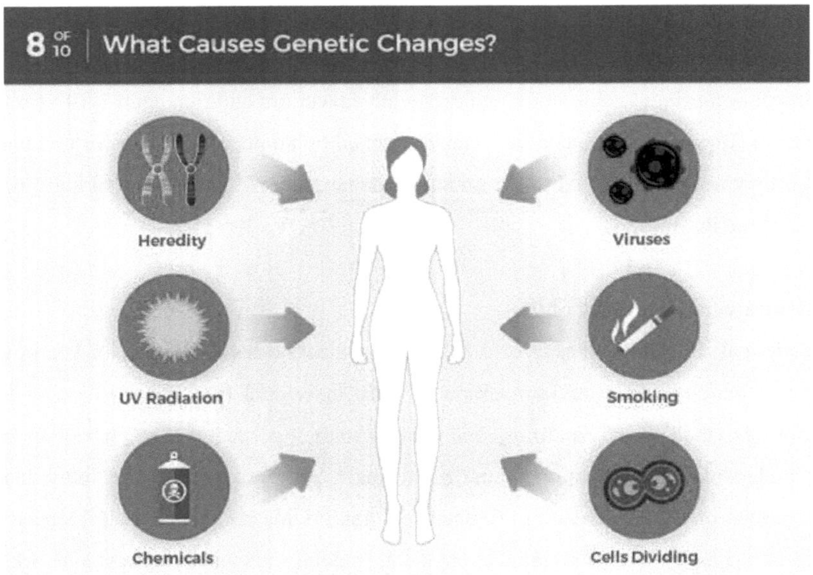

Figure 33. What Is Cancer?

4) Quality of life specific to children with cancer

Theoretical definition: A general sense of well-being based on the ability to participate in routine activities, interact with others, and adapt to disturbing cognitive, emotional, and physical events, and to create a sense of illness.

Practical definition: In this study, we mean the total points that the mothers of the studied units obtain from answering the questions of the specific questionnaire of cancer patients. This questionnaire includes 5 dimensions of therapeutic complications: pain or injury (two cases) and nausea (five cases), psychological: anxiety (three cases) and perception of physical appearance (three cases), emotional: anxiety when performing diagnostic procedures (three cases) And treatment anxiety (three cases), social: communication (three cases), cognitive: cognitive problems (three cases) and examines the quality of life associated with the disease in children and adolescents 2-18 years of age cancer. The score of this questionnaire is 5 points in Likert method and a score higher than the average is a sign of good quality of life.

5) Individual _social factors

Theoretical definition: Factors related to a person's personal characteristics that include a person's demographic characteristics. Demographic characteristics are a set of special moods, qualities, and characteristics that distinguish one person from others.

Practical definition: In this study, the meaning of individual-social factors is: child age, child gender, parent age, parent education, parental employment status, child living conditions, average monthly income, health insurance status and type It is the place of residence, the number of family members and the use of social support systems.

6) Clinical factors

Theoretical definition: disease-related factors according to studies including type of cancer, duration of disease, duration of treatment, type of treatment, is the distance between chemotherapy courses and the number of radiation therapy courses.

Practical definition: Factors related to the disease is the theoretical definition that after the interview with the mother, the intensity of each relationship will be measured using a regression model.

7) General health

Theoretical definition: It is a quality of life that is related to the sum of mental, spiritual and biological fitness of the person and adapts the person to his environment and enables him to perform a sufficient amount of physical-psychological and social activities.

Practical definition: General health of mothers of the studied units was obtained from the total score obtained to the questions raised in the General Health Questionnaire

(GHQ) of 12 Goldberg cases and based on it to three levels (0_12), partially desirable (13_24) and undesirable (25_36) is reported. (Discussed in detail in the data collection tool)

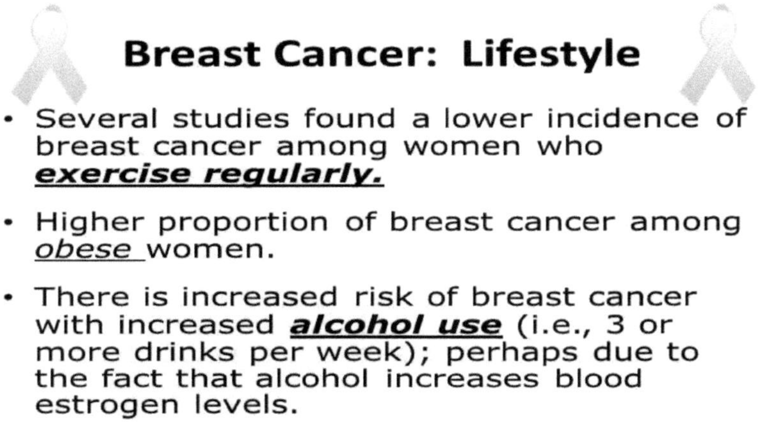

Breast Cancer: Lifestyle

- Several studies found a lower incidence of breast cancer among women who ***exercise regularly.***

- Higher proportion of breast cancer among *obese* women.

- There is increased risk of breast cancer with increased ***alcohol use*** (i.e., 3 or more drinks per week); perhaps due to the fact that alcohol increases blood estrogen levels.

Figure 34. You only get one body, Take good care of it

Research limitations

In this study, the quality-of-life interview was conducted when the children came with the mother because of a problem or for treatment, in which case it was somewhat difficult to complete a tool that had multiple questionnaires and many questions. On the other hand, due to the fact that the questionnaire used was a report by the mother and the quality of life related to children's health and specificity was evaluated during the past month, mothers may have difficulty or hesitation in remembering issues.

Research framework

The framework of this research is a concept based on the concept of pediatric cancer and quality of life. In this regard, the definition, epidemiology and types of cancer, clinical manifestations, diagnostic methods, treatment and complications, definition of quality of life and its areas, measurement methods Quality of life, factors related to quality of life are discussed.

Despite advances in the control and prevention of infectious diseases in recent decades, the incidence of chronic diseases has increased. Chronic disease affects all stages of life. Although some diseases have little effect on quality of life, most of them have significant effects on the quality of life due to the disability they leave behind. One of the special features of these diseases is their long-term nature or the uncertainty of the course of the disease. Therefore, in addition to a lot of effort for treatment, it also requires a lot of costs. Among the disorders that severely affect the health and consequently the quality of life of individuals are chronic diseases such as cancer which is considered as one of the most important health problems in communities. Its prevalence has increased among chronic non-communicable diseases.

Smardak believes that cancer is now a life-threatening chronic disease. The first evidence of cancer dates back to 1500 BC, when it was discovered by a German archaeologist named Ebres in 1873 during an excavation in Egypt. "Arsenic pastes are effective in improving them." The wise Hippocrates identified several cancerous tumors in 500 BC, and in the second century AD, Galen discussed the cause of cancer. Bu Ali Sina, a great Iranian physician, studied cancer in the 10th century, and in 1761 Morgan founded a new pathology and described cancer.

Cancer occurs when a specific cell of cells begins to multiply and grow uncontrollably so that normal cells are reduced. In some countries, cancer is the second leading cause of death after cardiovascular disease. But in Iran, after cardiovascular disease and accidents, cancer is the third leading cause of death. The disease is also seen in children. Cancer is one of the leading causes of death among children. In the United States and Australia, it is the second leading cause of death among children aged 0 to 14 years after unintentional injuries.

Childhood neoplasms include various types of malignant tumors called cancers and non-malignant tumors. Children, like adults, can get cancer in any part of the body, but some types of cancer are more common in children. There are several types of cancer in children, including leukemia, brain cancer, lymphoma, Hodgkin's disease, Wilms' tumor, neuroblastoma, osteosarcoma, Ewing sarcoma, retinoblastoma, and rhabdomyosarcoma ", of which leukemia is the most common cancer. It is a childhood period.

Leukemia is a broad term used to refer to a group of malignant diseases of the bone marrow and lymphatic system and is the most common malignant neoplasm of childhood and adolescence, accounting for about 31% of all malignancies in children under 15 years of age. Leukemia is a cancer of the white blood cells. The cancer starts in the bone marrow, but then spreads to the lymph nodes, spleen, liver, central nervous system, or other organs. The most common type of childhood leukemia is acute lymphoblastic leukemia, which accounts for 77% of all childhood cancers. It is more common in whites and in boys. Subgroups of acute myelogenous leukemia account for 11% and chronic myelogenous leukemia less than 3%, and other chronic myelomonocytic leukemia and chronic lymphocytic leukemia in childhood account for 1 to 2% of cases. The most common general symptoms of acute lymphoblastic leukemia are fever, anemia, paleness, fatigue, weakness, recurrent infections, and bone pain.

The second most common group of cancers in children is brain tumors. Brain tumors are classified and named based on the tissue in which they spread. Brain tumors can occur at any age, even in infants and adults. Approximately 2,200 primary brain tumors are diagnosed in children and adolescents each year, with a total annual incidence of 28 per million children under the age of 19. This type of cancer will have different early manifestations depending on the location, type, rate of tumor growth and age of the child. Signs and symptoms are related to obstruction of cerebrospinal fluid flow. Tumors located above the tentacle present as mild personality, mental, and speech changes. In young children, open cranial sutures may present with common signs of increased intracranial pressure, such as vomiting, drowsiness, and restlessness, as well as late findings of macrocephaly. It is often difficult to diagnose this type of cancer because the symptoms are often seen in many physical and mental disorders.

RISK FACTORS
OF PROSTATE CANCER:

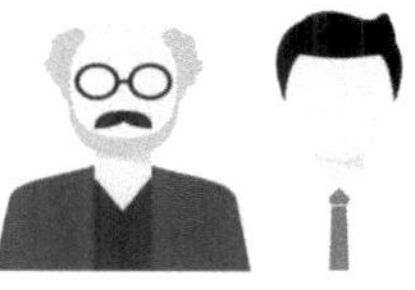

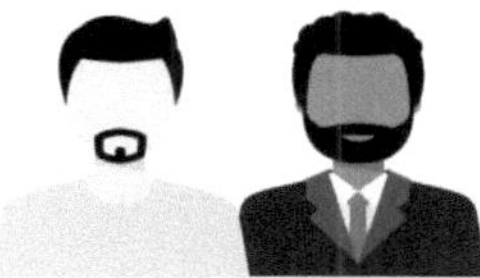

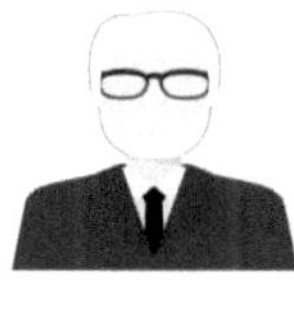

AGE
The risk of prostate cancer increases with age, especially **after the age of 50**.

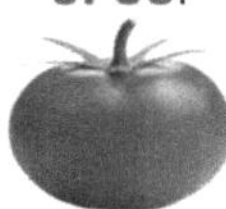

FAMILY HISTORY
If you have a **first degree relative** – father, brother or son – with prostate cancer, the risk of developing prostate cancer is 2 to 3 times higher than the average risk.

RACE/ ETHNICITY
Prostate cancer is increasing among **Asian men** in urbanized environment, particularly those who have a lifestyle with **less physical activity** and **less healthy diet**.

Figure 35. Six Things You Need to Know About Prostate Cancer

Another common cancer in children is lymphoma, which develops in lymph tissues such as the lymph nodes, spleen, and thymus, which produce and store infection-fighting cells. Lymphoma is the third most common childhood cancer in the United States, with an annual incidence of 15 cases per million children under the age of 14. Lymphoma is generally divided into "Hodgkin" and "non-Hodgkin" diseases. Hodgkin's disease involves most of the peripheral lymph nodes (those close to the surface of the body), the first sign of which is a painless bulge in the neck, armpits, or groin. Non-Hodgkin's lymphoma is also more common in children, especially in the gut, near the appendix, and may be seen in the upper chest.

Symptoms include abnormal pain or swelling, difficulty breathing, and sometimes difficulty swallowing or swelling of the face and neck. It may also occur in other organs such as the liver, spleen, bone marrow, lymph nodes, nervous system and bones.

Wilms' tumor is the most common intra-abdominal and renal tumor in children. It is a cancer that originates from kidney cells and is seen in children from infancy to 15 years of age and rarely in older ages and is different from kidney cancers in adults. Approximately 95% of children with kidney cancer have Wilms-type tumors. About 6% of common cancers in children are Wilms' tumors. The most common age for Wilms's tumor is in the first five years of life, usually between the ages of three and four. Girls are more likely to get it than boys. This type of cancer can be inherited and affects both kidneys in about 5% of cases. Parents usually take their child to the doctor after seeing a small bulge in the abdomen. Symptoms such as blood in the urine, weakness, fever, loss of appetite, or abdominal pain may also be present.

Neuroblastoma is a type of cancer of the peripheral sympathetic system that is seen in infants and children and rarely in adults. It accounts for about 8% of childhood malignancies. Cells of this type of cancer are usually the primary and developing neurons found in the embryo or fetus. More than half of neuroblastoma tumors occur in the adrenal glands, located in the abdominal cavity and near the kidneys. Neuroblastoma may occur anywhere in the sympathetic nerve tissue. Signs and symptoms of neuroblastoma indicate the location of the tumor and the extent of the disease. Nervous signs and symptoms are the first manifestation of the disease.

Retinoblastoma is a rare eye cancer that may be inherited and affects both eyes in a third of cases. It can often be seen by looking into the eyes of young people. But it is usually diagnosed by examination under general anesthesia. This type of cancer tends to stay local for a long time, but in advanced stages, it may spread to other parts of the body.

Osteosarcoma is the most common bone cancer in children. The riskiest period for osteosarcoma is the growth spurt of puberty. This suggests a link between rapid bone growth and malignancy. Children with this type of cancer usually complain of pain or swelling. The disease is difficult to diagnose because it is easily confused with local infections, defects and disorders of the secretory glands, arthritis, vitamin deficiencies and harmless tumors. Osteosarcoma usually spreads to other parts of the body, especially the lungs.

Ewing sarcoma, which is actually undifferentiated bone sarcoma, may also originate in soft tissue. It is more common in men than women and often spreads to other bones and lungs. The symptoms of Ewing sarcoma are similar to those of osteosarcoma. Common symptoms of the disease include pain, swelling, limited mobility and tenderness of bone or soft tissue, fever, and weight loss.

Rhabdomyosarcoma, also called rhabdomyosarcoma, originates from muscle cells. It most often affects males and children between the ages of 2 and 6. Although the disease can occur in any muscle tissue, it is most commonly found in the head and neck, pelvis, and extremities. The most common clinical manifestation is a mass that may be painful or painless. Symptoms of the disease are due to displacement or obstruction of the body's natural structures.

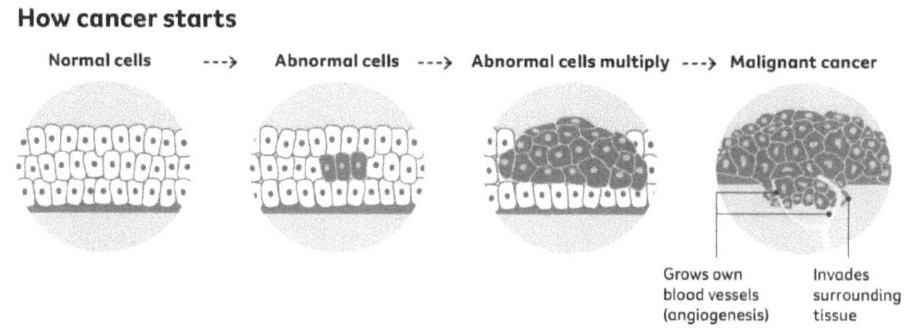

Figure 36. What is cancer? Cancer Council Victoria

Although the underlying cause of cancer is unknown, some cancers can be attributed to a genetic defect. Children with chromosomal abnormalities or immune deficiencies are at risk for a variety of cancers. Other factors associated with the increased incidence of cancer are exposure to environmental factors that can lead to gene mutations at any stage of cell division and predispose a person to cancer. So that contact with environmental factors in a susceptible person may be the main cause of childhood cancer. Rapid growth and development in infants and children make them more exposed to these factors. Given these cases, environmental risk factors and extensive chromosomal defects and immunodeficiency syndromes are important diseases that must be carefully identified and tracked in children.

Proper diagnosis and staging of the disease is necessary, especially for childhood cancers with a high cure rate, because the type of treatment depends on the type of cancer. Proper and accurate staging of the disease reduces the risk of acute and severe side effects and long-term treatment problems in patients with a prognosis that requires less treatment to achieve full recovery. Diagnostic imaging techniques are a very important step in further evaluating children with solid tumors. MRI, CT scan, ultrasonography, scintigraphy, spectroscopy is useful in the evaluation of children with cancer if they are used properly.

During treatment, the effectiveness of treatment and the rate of improvement in response to treatment in many pediatric cancers are evaluated using imaging techniques. Diagnostic, laboratory, and pathological methods are vital in diagnosing and treating children with cancer.

Today, with the development of medical science and related technology, cancer has gradually changed from a deadly and acute disease to a chronic disease and their survival rate has increased. In contrast to the annual increase of one percent in cancer incidence, the number of successful treatments for this disease has increased by 0.25 percent each year. In 2003, Canada also found that the survival of children with cancer had increased over the past 30 years as a result of using a combination of aggressive drugs. In 2000, the survival rate of children with cancer was reported to be 60%. At present, in Iran, with the improvement of social, economic and health care status, 70% of children with cancer survive for more than 5 years.

Treating children with cancer is one of the most complex efforts in pediatrics. Therapeutic goals are presented to the cancer patient based on the specific realistic and achievable goals of each type of cancer. Complete eradication of malignant disease, long-term survival and inhibition of cancer cell growth (control) and elimination of disease-related symptoms (relief) are possible goals of treatment. Depending on the type of cancer, children are treated with invasive and combination therapies of chemotherapy, radiotherapy and surgery. More than two treatments are often used together.

The most widely used treatment for children with cancer is chemotherapy. Combination therapy is almost always used. Most cytotoxic drugs used for childhood cancers are selected from a variety of drug groups, including alkylating agents, antibodies, antibiotics, hormones, plant alkaloids, and topoisomerase inhibitors. Their side effects generally affect the proliferation of all cell populations. Most tissues and organs that have a rapid cell cycle, such as bone marrow, oral and intestinal mucosa, epidermis, liver, and sperm tissue, are vulnerable. Bone marrow suppression (along with neutropenia and thrombocytopenia, which are the most common problems), immune suppression, nausea and vomiting, liver dysfunction, gastrointestinal mucositis, dermatitis, and hair loss are the most common acute side effects of these drugs.

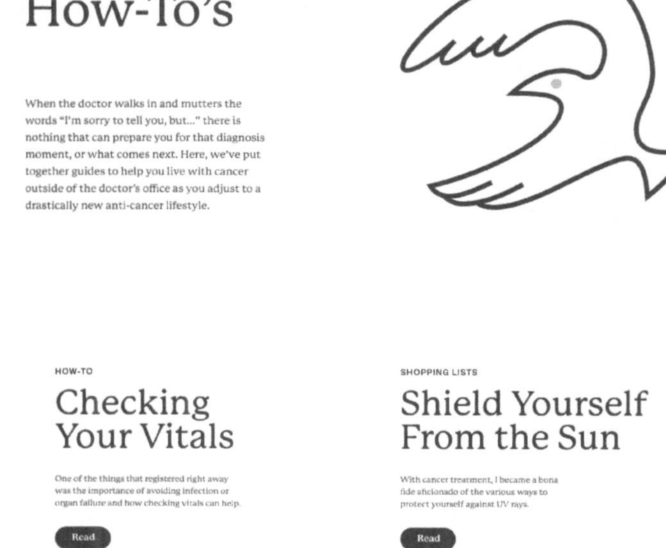

Figure 37. The Platform for Cancer Patients

In a study of the side effects of chemotherapy in adolescents, 59 percent said the side effects of anti-cancer therapies were worse than the cancer itself. The physical and psychological effects of chemotherapy in patients cause fear of starting chemotherapy and even resistance or rejection of anti-cancer treatment programs. In addition, it imposes high costs on patients and the health care network, such as longer hospital stays, increased nursing and medical costs, and reduced patients' quality of life and performance.

Radiation therapy is another way to treat cancer in which ionizing radiation to cancer cells prevents the cells from multiplying and killing them. Radiation therapy may have a palliative aspect (to prevent further cancer growth) or a therapeutic aspect (to eradicate the disease). In children, who are more vulnerable to the side effects of ionizing radiation than adults, cautious radiation is used. A major breakthrough in pediatric radiation therapy has been the use of adaptive radiation in children with cancer. This method is generally used as radiation therapy with moderate intensity and does not reach the normal tissues of the radiation by adapting the volume of the radiation to the shape of the tumor. Side effects of radiation therapy depend on the amount of radiation given to the person and the area of the body that has been exposed to the radiation. Like chemotherapy, most tissues and organs that have a rapid cell cycle are vulnerable.

Most children with cancer need surgery during their treatment. For example, determining the tumor's response to treatment, inserting a central venous catheter, sampling to diagnose a tumor, or removing solid tumors from surgery are used. The use of surgery increases the risk of adhesions. The negative effect of surgery depends on the area and extent of surgery.

Although severe treatment of childhood cancers can increase the survival of affected children, it can also lead to increased late complications, adverse changes, and recurrence of the disease process. Almost no organ is immune in the treatment process, and often all anti-cancer substances, especially radiation, are responsible for some harmful effects and results. The most devastating late complication is the development of secondary malignancy. Children under 5 years of age who have undergone cranial radiation therapy are more prone to developing brain tumors. Anthracycline treatment is associated with cardiomyopathy. Cranial irradiation and spinal chemotherapy are associated with emotional and neuropsychological problems that are only part of the long-term consequences of the disease.

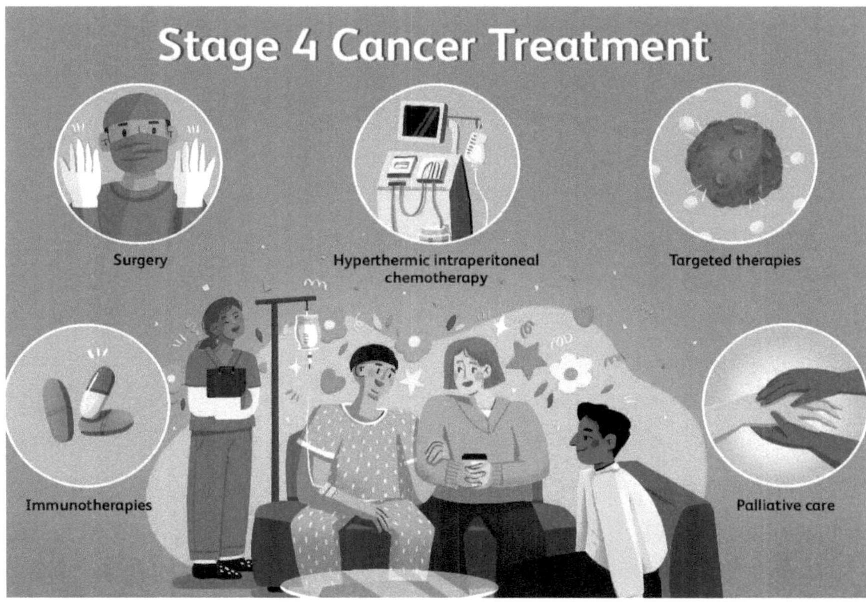

Figure 38. Stage 4 Cancer: Definition, Diagnosis, Treatment

Various studies have shown that the presence of a chronic disease such as cancer and subsequent, long-term and invasive treatments such as chemotherapy and radiation in addition to the above-mentioned physical effects affect various aspects of the patient's life and reduce his quality of life. For example, psychological stress and anxiety are other common consequences after the diagnosis of cancer that psychological and social dimensions threaten the quality of life of these children. These stresses vary for parents and children during different stages of cancer, including diagnosis, treatment, remission, and survival after treatment. Cancer is a disease that changes the course of a person's life. A person with cancer cannot continue to live as in the past and for almost all people with cancer, it creates many problems in all aspects of personal and social life and causes feelings of dependence, decreased self-esteem, increased feelings of vulnerability and confusion.

Pain, physical symptoms and overall decline in quality of life. Adverse physiological conditions of cancer patients such as anorexia, nausea, vomiting, sensory changes and electrolytes in the body and stress caused by cancer affect their quality of life and physical function. Also, treatment of most cancers has toxicity and side effects that severely endanger the short-term and long-term quality of life of patients. Obviously, awareness of quality of life can improve the quality of life of a child with cancer. In this regard, efforts to measure the quality of life for cancer patients began in 1940.

Today, due to the epidemiological change of acute diseases to chronic types, the quantity of life, which was measured by criteria such as mortality, has become less important and attention has been paid to a new component called quality of life that affects the disease and therapeutic interventions. Measures the patient's daily life. Major advances in public health and preventive medicine have led to a revision of the definition of health, perhaps the most important of which is the use of quality of life.

Historically, quality of life has been introduced as a concept in Greek philosophy. At that time, Aristotle considered "good life" or "doing good things" to mean happiness, but at the same time he mentioned the difference between the concept of happiness in different people and mentioned that health causes happiness in a sick person. It is not the same with wealth that makes a poor person happy, and it has clearly stated that happiness not only has different meanings for different people but also does not have the same meaning for a person in different circumstances.

Research on quality of life was developed in the 1970s to examine the impact of different conditions on people's daily lives, to assess their emotional and social performance, as well as their physical performance. The application of this concept to measure the impact of disease and therapies on people's lives and their performance in various aspects of life led to the development of a field of research called quality of life related to health. Quality of life assessments usually work better than traditional and clinical assessments of the emotional and social consequences of disease progression and treatment.

As mentioned, quality of life is used to assess the general health status of individuals and communities. In fact, since 1984, when the World Health Organization declared that health is not just the absence of disease, but a state of complete physical, mental and social well-being, experts' attention has been drawn to the importance of quality of life. There are many definitions of quality of life.

The theoretical definition offered for quality of life is: a combination of physical, mental, social well-being that is perceived by an individual or a group of people. Such as: satisfaction, expectations, health and economic status. The issue of quality of life is very important in different groups, especially those who have special physical, mental and psychological conditions or face the stresses caused by those special conditions. The term is used in a wide range of fields, including international development, health care, and political science.

Quality of life should not be used instead of standard of living because quality of life, in addition to income, includes other aspects of life such as home environment, physical and mental health, education and social affiliation. In other words, quality of life is a logical process and a concept based on culture, which shows a summary of the values, beliefs, symbols and experiences formed by that culture and a way to know and understand human conditions and experiences in life. Provide. Therefore, quality of life is a powerful force in guiding, maintaining and promoting health and wellness in different societies and cultures.

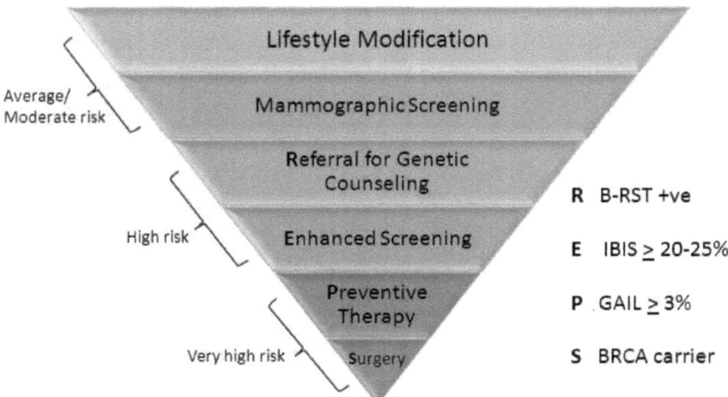

Figure 39. Breast Cancer Screening and Diagnosis

Regarding the quality of life, Fassino says that quality of life is a key indicator today, and since quality of life includes many dimensions such as physiological aspects and performance of the individual, it is important to pay attention to it and to evaluate it correctly. Quality of life should pay attention to the above dimensions. Although there is no general agreement on the definition of quality of life, but the important characteristics of quality of life that are often agreed upon by most experts in the humanities and social sciences are its multidimensionality, subjectivity and dynamism. The dynamic nature of quality of life helps researchers to provide better contexts for people by conducting research on quality-of-life strategies. Being multidimensional means different dimensions that are raised in the quality of life and being mental means mental and value traits in the life of each person that affect his attitude towards life. Liu concluded in a study that quality of life includes two important components, mental (psychological) and objective (social, economic, political and environmental). Subjective items are mostly qualitative in nature and are generally individual and not measurable, while objective items are more quantitative and measurable. Initial studies on health concepts did not pay attention to patients' opinions. As a result, these studies were not acceptable to patients. Today, however, self-assessment of patients' health status is part of the assessment process.

In fact, the concept of quality of life is used to refer to objective conditions and mental recovery. This means that a good quality of life is created by good physical health and support from family and friends, as well as a person's sense of happiness and satisfaction. Undoubtedly, external objective factors such as income and longevity affect the quality of life. Contrary to this view, some believe that quality of life is a mental assessment of life satisfaction, and some combine a person's mental assessment of well-being with physical symptoms, job performance, sexual function, emotional status, and so on. Diseases can change the patient's assessment of health and quality of life by causing physical, social, economic, etc. disruption.

Quality of life is an important criterion that shows the effectiveness of health care, level of health and sense of well-being and makes it possible to predict the occurrence of mortality and the rate of hospitalization of the patient. Over the last 20 years, the interest in evaluating and improving the quality of life of patients with chronic diseases has increased significantly, and improving the daily functioning and quality of life of patients with chronic diseases has become a goal. The primary goal of treatment, especially in chronic disease, is to enhance the quality of life by reducing the effects of the disease, and patients with severe and chronic diseases should not necessarily have a low quality of life. Members of the healthcare team can influence the quality of life of patients by monitoring their health status or improving it. Also, by measuring the quality of life, the negative impact of the disease on the quality of life can be determined.

In medical sciences, in particular, measuring the quality of life has the following applications: a) determining the effectiveness of various treatments, b) evaluating health services and prioritizing them, c) policy-making and resource allocation, d) improving physician-patient relationships by increasing Mutual understanding of the disease and its treatment, e) Research: During the last few decades, many researches on quality of life based on demographic indicators (such as age groups, gender, race, urban and rural social areas, social class, etc.) , Different cultures (at regional, national and regional level), time (longitudinal and cross-sectional studies), different organizational environments, etc., but what has recently been welcomed in the field of medical sciences, Evaluation of quality of life in certain groups of patients.

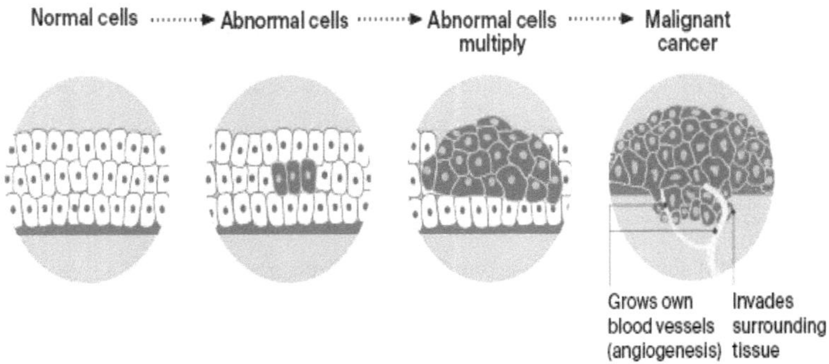

Figure 40. What is cancer?

Assessing the quality of life in health studies is important in that it is an auxiliary measure in measuring the recovery of patients and also a helpful method in evaluating the results of various treatments and thus by assessing the quality of life of patients and identifying the effects of the disease on the dimensions. Different ways of life can be used more appropriate treatment methods and evaluate the treatment results in a short time and try to improve it and can also provide useful factors about the components of life and it can be measured by a numerical score. The title expressed the quality of life score. In the past, quality of life measuring instruments were mostly used to assess the physical condition of patients, but today it is often used for different emotional aspects and beliefs of people.

Comprehensive tools, especially those that measure health symptoms, are useful and effective in providing information about the functional state of health. Tools are available to assess health-related quality of life, such as quality of life questionnaires for young children, school-age children, adults translated into English and other languages. Most of the items in these tools are grouped around two questions:

1- Health problems in the past few weeks,

2- Emotional reactions to problems. The questions are divided to cover all aspects of health-related quality of life.

The tools used in research are general or specific. Using general tools, quality of life can be measured on a large scale in different groups of patients such as heart, lung, vascular, AIDS and cancer patients or healthy people using a questionnaire and compared with each other. This type of tool will be crucial, especially in cases where people are not sick but the quality of life is low for various reasons. Specific tools can only be used for specific diseases or specific groups of people. Specific tools include items related to the symptoms of the disease (pain, arthritis) or the side effects of treatment (nausea in cancer). The disadvantage of this group of tools is that it is not possible to compare between different groups and in general these tools are not as complete as general tools, instead they are more sensitive and responsive.

It is necessary to evaluate the quality of life in cancer patients and determine the factors affecting their quality of life, because the factors affecting the quality of life in patients with cancer are not only physiological changes during the disease but also the mental state. Psychologically, a person's reaction to the results of diagnostic tests also depends on the prognosis of the disease and the stages of sadness, grief and anger. Quality of life in cancer patients is affected by individual social and clinical factors. As a result, there are many factors that can potentially reduce the quality of life of cancer patients. By identifying these factors and cases that increase the symptoms of depression and anxiety in cancer patients, we can improve the quality of life of these patients in the short and long term. For example, cancer-related factors such as the type of cancer, the type of treatment, and the characteristics of the cancer include: fatigue, mental health problems, denial of the disease, mental imbalance due to changes in organ function, and duration of illness on quality of life.

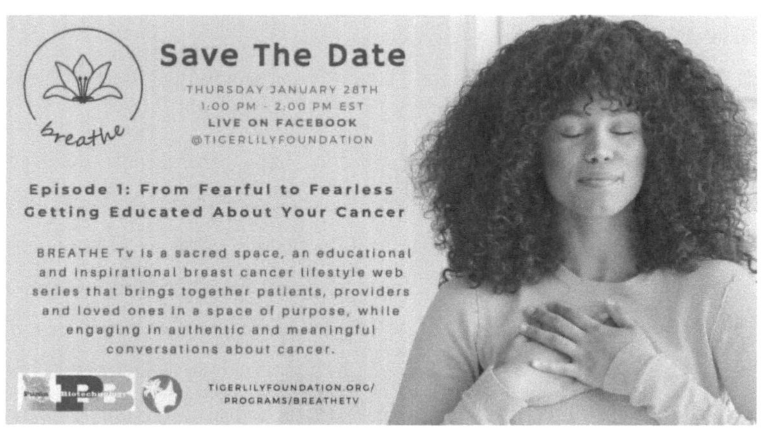

Figure 41. Getting Educated About Your Cancer

Other factors such as the severity of the disease, psychological stress as well as the stage of the disease can affect the quality of life of cancer patients. The quality of life of people with chronic diseases is related to their individual characteristics and, in fact, depends on the adaptation skills of people in different life situations to what they have already learned about self-control. Therefore, their responses to different life situations are different and physical illness is one of the situations that affect these responses. Studies have shown that low levels of education, lack of jobs and low incomes reduce the quality of life. Therefore, individual and social factors are more important in people with chronic diseases than in healthy people.

In addition to the adverse effects of cancer on a child's quality of life, the mental and physical health of parents is also affected. Frequent hospitalization, unpredictability of the course of the disease, changes in the physical condition of the sick child and the emergence of complications from the disease and treatment, cause severe depression of parents, especially in the first months after diagnosis. Parents whose children are being treated for cancer, especially if the severity of the treatment is severe and the child is in poor health and has not been diagnosed for a long time, are more anxious so that the emotional and psychological functioning of the parents is affected by the mental functioning of the child. Parents who are more stressed are more likely to have a lot of stress with their children, and vice versa. As a result, there is a relationship between the consequences of parent-child stress and they affect each other's performance. Especially the negative performance of the child can adversely affect the psychological adjustment of his parents.

Children who have more behavioral and emotional problems cause more psychological problems in their mothers. When a child becomes ill, the mother becomes more involved in caring for the child than the father and takes more responsibility for treatment and decision making. Instead, the father tends to do work and try to keep calm in other family members.

These differences cause mothers to experience many changes in their lives and lose their jobs or work short hours due to staying with their child in the hospital. Other factors that cause psychological stress in mothers, such as: Lack of information about the disease and low knowledge to help the child adapt to recent situations, which can be reduced through psychological examinations and interviews, psychological stress of parents and Increased adjustment and reduced child psychological problems because cancer is a chronic disease that affects the family during treatment. The family must constantly adapt to the changes that are taking place in the field of disease and cancer treatment.

Nurses by explaining about the disease and treatment, emotional support, helping to investigate and identify the causes of stress, recommending the use of coping mechanisms and problem-solving methods, continuing efforts to meet evolutionary needs and spiritual beliefs, in coping with the disease can be effective. Since nurses and other members of the flagship treatment team are changing to promote health among the community, they are obliged to provide the information needed by parents of children with cancer, because lack of parental knowledge and awareness can affect parental performance. Parents' interaction with the child and the quality of life of the sick child have a negative impact. Also, one of the key and important tasks of oncology nurses is to prevent, identify and control the complications of cancer and its treatment, which has an important effect on improving the quality of life of patients and accelerating their recovery. By identifying different aspects of patients 'lives, nurses not only try to mitigate these problems, but also by providing problems to relevant social organizations and patients' families, they can attract the necessary cooperation to improve the quality of life.

In this regard, health care providers and researchers in the first step should obtain more information about the quality of life of these patients and how to improve it, and by taking effective decisions and measures based on the findings of this study to improve the quality of life of children with cancer.

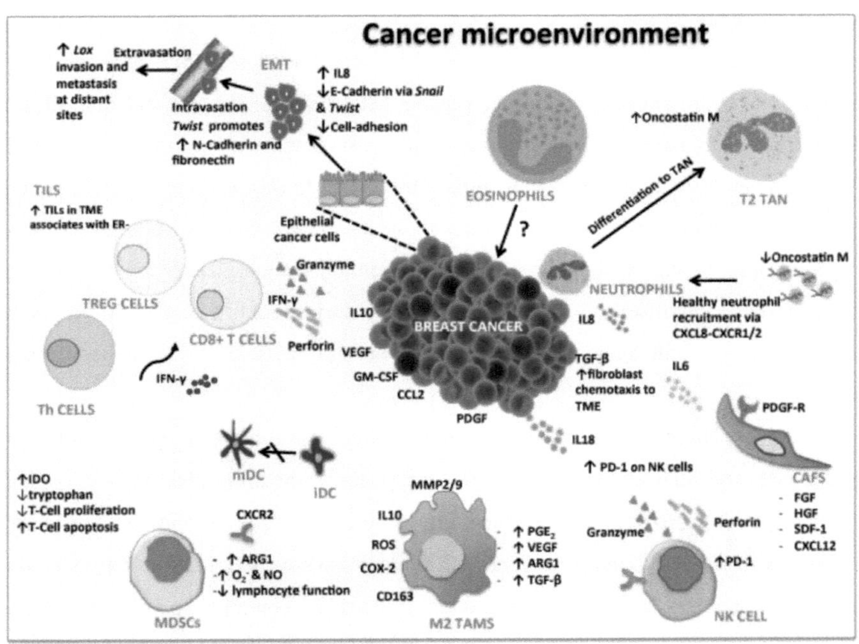

Figure 42. Cancer immunology

Chapter V

Literature review

Due to the importance of quality of life in cancer patients, the study of cancer has gone beyond the traditional medical implications and the effects of the disease on the quality of life of patients have been included. Quality of life is defined as a multidimensional structure and includes patients' perceptions of the disease and the effect of the disease and treatment on various aspects of life, including physical, mental and social functions. So far, several studies have been conducted in different countries on the quality of life of children with cancer in nursing. The results of some studies showed an association between disease, treatment, individual-social and clinical factors in the areas of children's quality of life, and some other studies did not. In this research, 9 articles related to the research topic are discussed.

Increasing the survival of children with cancer has emphasized the importance of health and quality of life in these children. In this regard, Morris et al. (2008) conducted a longitudinal study entitled Health-Related Quality of Life in Young Children with Out-of-Central Nervous Cancer After Successful Treatment in Amsterdam.

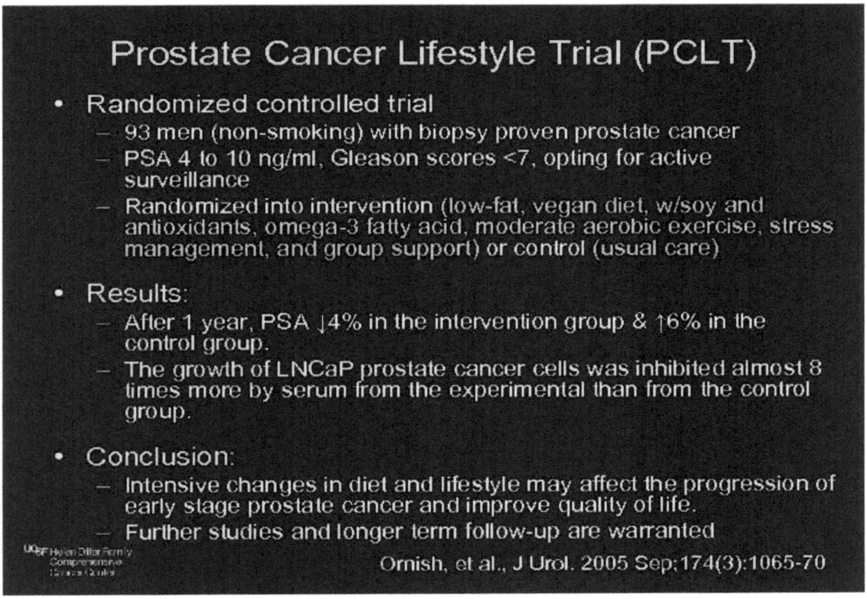

Figure 43. Nutrition Prostate Cancer Exploring the role

The questions of this study include: 1) What is the quality of life related to the health of young healers during the first three years after successful treatment? 2) To what extent are the clinical variables, demographics and psychological stress of parents related to the quality of life related to the health of young healers? Parents of 53 young children who had been successfully treated for the disease participated in the study. In order to collect data, the quality-of-life questionnaire of young children in the age range of 1-5 years was used, which measured the child's performance in 6 dimensions:

1- Physical function including: sleep, appetite, lung, stomach, skin,

2- Motor function including: activities Motor;

3- Examines social functioning including: communication, behavioral issues,

4- Cognitive function including: cognitive problems,

5- Negative moods including: anxiety,

6- Positive moods including: positive mood, vitality.

This questionnaire is completed by the parents and they evaluate the questions related to the events of the last month. The scoring of this questionnaire is done in 5 points by Likert method. Thus, for positive mood and vitality: the option is always 0 points, the option is often 1 point, the option is sometimes 2 points, the option is rarely 3 points and the option is never 4 points, and for other dimensions the option is never 0 points and the option is always 4 points. Then the scores are reversed and converted to 0_100 (0 = 100, 1 = 75, 2 = 50, 3 = 25, 0 = 4). Then the percentage of points obtained and the average percentage in each dimension is calculated that the higher the score, the better the quality of life. These studies were performed at 2 months, 1 year, 2 years, 3 years after the end of treatment. A 30-item general health questionnaire was used to assess parents' psychological stress.

A higher score indicated greater psychological stress. SPSS version 12 was used to analyze all data. Linear regression statistical method was used to predict the variables related to quality of life. The results showed that the quality of life of children with cancer, two months after treatment, had a worse score compared to the healthy group (p <0.001), healed in the areas of behavior, anxiety, motor function, positive mood and sleep. They reported bad scores. One year after treatment, compared with the healthy group, the quality of life associated with the health of the recovered improved significantly, but there was still anxiety (p <0.01) and difficulty in motor function (p <0.001). The level of health-related quality of life was normal in years 2 and 3, and the healers were no different from the healthy group. The course of treatment, the poor prognosis, and the severe psychological stress of the parents resulted in a worse score in the physical dimension of quality of life. According to the data, it is concluded that young children adapt well to the experience of cancer, so that at the end of treatment, the quality of life related to health is significantly improved.

In this regard, for children aged 6-15 years, another study by Landolt et al. (2006) is a prospective study, with the aim of assessing health-related quality of life in children with cancer during the first year after cancer diagnosis and comparison with healthy children.

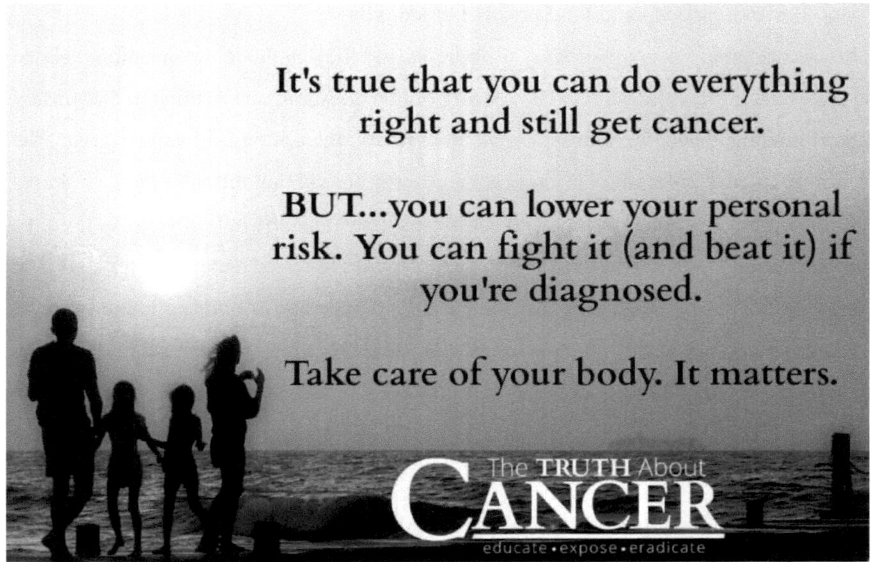

Figure 44. Cancer – Why Some Get It and Some Don't

The relationship between health-related quality of life and parental characteristics, treatment, illness, economic status, and demographics was determined in Germany.

Inclusion criteria include: have recently been diagnosed with cancer, are between 6-15 years old, have no disease other than cancer, are fluent in German, and do not have mental retardation. Fifty-two sick children, aged 6-15 years, participated in the study with their parents. Examinations were performed six weeks and one year after diagnosis. Demographic information of the child and parents was obtained through interviews with parents and information related to the disease from the records of these patients and was also graded by the oncologist, the course of treatment and the functional status of the child.

The severity of treatment, drug side effects and functional status of the child were divided into three parts: severity of treatment:

1 = low severity (surgery alone or six months of chemotherapy alone or both with a good prognosis),

2 = moderate severity (Treatment longer than six months with a moderate prognosis (such as osteosarcoma),

3 = high severity (high-risk treatments such as bone marrow transplantation with an unfavorable prognosis), as well as classification of drug side effects:

0 = no side effects,

1 = moderate side effects (Such as hospitalization, infection),

2 = severe complications (failure to respond to treatment, frequent hospitalizations) and functional status of the child:

0 = good functional status,

1 = moderate functional status,

2 = poor functional status done.

The TACQL Children's General Quality of Life Questionnaire was used to assess health-related quality of life. This tool has seven dimensions (physical, independent activities, social activities, cognitive activities, motor activities, positive moods and negative moods) and each dimension is composed of eight subgroups. The scoring of this questionnaire is done in 5 points by Likert method.

Due to the increasing survival rate of children with cancer, attention to their psychological, social and educational needs is important and should be one of the goals of treatment and care of these patients.

In this regard, Munir et al. (2007), a study aimed at: 1) determining the quality of life of school-age children in the field of social, emotional and physical performance, 2) identifying predictors of quality of life and 3) describing educational achievements among children They did a school for cancer in Alexandria (in Egypt). 215 school-age children with cancer who went to outpatient centers for treatment participated in the study.

Quality of life tools of children with cancer were used to collect data. Demographic information such as: age, gender, socio-economic status, education and occupation of parents, household income was collected through a researcher-made questionnaire through interviews with parents.

The socio-economic level of the family was determined based on the scores of the comprehension system and L_Sherbani (1983). Scores range from 5 to 19. Scores higher than 15 (more than 80% of the score) were at the high level, scores above 11_14 (between 60 and 80% of the score) were at the intermediate level, and scores below 11 (less than 60% of the score) were at the lower socio-economic level. In order to estimate the educational achievements, the students' grade point average of the previous year was evaluated. Clinical factors including: tumor type, time of diagnosis, duration of disease and complications of treatment were extracted from patients' records. After coding, the data were entered into SPSS software version 10.

Descriptive statistics such as mean and standard deviation and inferential statistics of Chi-square, ANOVA, Mann-Whitney and multiple regression analysis were used. The results of the study showed that lymphoma (34.9%) was the most common type of cancer, followed by leukemia (24.2%), brain tumor (13%), osteosarcoma (7.9%) and Wilms tumor (7%). They gave. The prevalence of lymphoma was higher among boys than girls (39.3% vs. 26.7%) while the prevalence of leukemia, brain tumor, osteosarcoma and Wilms tumor was higher among girls than boys) (xx = 56.56, 05 / 0 p <). 48% of girls and 30.7% of boys had poor quality of life (x2 = 7.39, p <0.05). Boys had a good quality of life in the physical dimension (p <0.01).

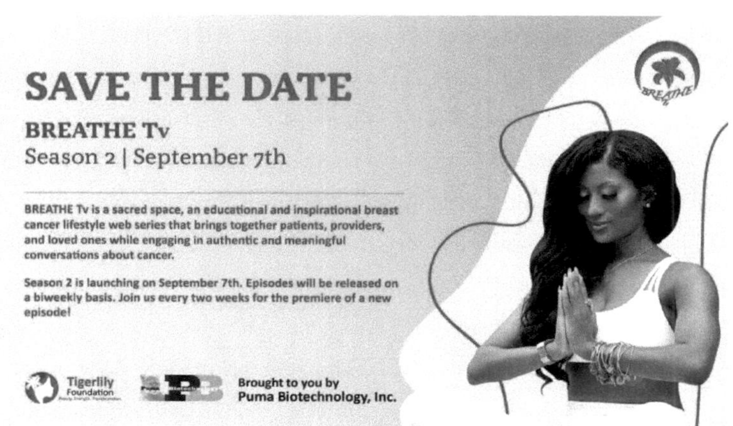

Figure 45. Tigerlily Foundation

The mean percentage of quality-of-life scores was significant among older patients (p = 0.04) and among boys (p = 0.03). The majority of patients (92.6%) were dissatisfied with the side effects of treatment and disease and their quality of life was significantly unsatisfactory (p <0.01) and also had a history of hospitalization. Educational achievements were reported as good and very good in 31.5% of cases and no difference was observed between the sexes (p> 0.05). Only age (p <0.01), side effects (p <0.01) and time of diagnosis (p <0.05) were significantly associated with quality of life. In the physical dimension, sex (p <0.05), age (p <0.05), side effects (p <0.01) and time of diagnosis (p <0.05) were predictors of poor quality of life. In the emotional dimension, age (p <0.01), side effects (p <0.01), time to start treatment (p <0.05) and time of diagnosis (p <0.05) were associated with low quality of life. In the social dimension, only the type of treatment (p <0.01) was related to quality of life. The results of this study suggest that health-related quality of life should be measured continuously in children with cancer in order to identify specific treatments that have fewer side effects and also to identify factors that affect their quality of life.

Cancer patients typically experience a range of symptoms, including pain and a variety of physical and mental disorders. Anxiety and other mood disorders may develop immediately after diagnosis, and these symptoms change over time in response to diagnosis, recurrence, and improvement of the disease. In this regard, Pack et al. (2010) conducted a prospective study in Singapore with the aim of 1) determining the quality of life of children with cancer and 2) identifying areas of quality of life that have been harmed by various treatments. Thirty-two children with cancer, aged 7 to 18, from the Pediatric Cancer Center in Singapore participated in the study. To collect data, the general questionnaire of children's quality of life and the specific questionnaire of quality of life of children with cancer were used. A dedicated questionnaire for cancer patients assesses the quality of life associated with the disease in children and adolescents aged 2-18 years with cancer. This tool has the following dimensions: a) Therapeutic complications include: pain or injuries, nausea b) Psychological including: worry, perception of physical appearance c) Emotional including: Anxiety when performing diagnostic procedures, Anxiety therapy d) Cognitive including: Cognitive problems c) Social includes: Communications are composed. Questions assess events from the past 1 month and are completed by children with cancer (Child Report Form). These questionnaires are scored in 5-point Likert style, so the option always has 4 points, often 3 points, sometimes 2 points, rarely 1 point and the option never has 0 points. Then the scores are reversed and converted to 0_100 (0 = 100, 1 = 75, 2 = 50, 3 = 25, 0 = 4). Then the percentage of points obtained and the average percentage in each dimension is calculated that the higher the score, the better the quality of life. The validity and reliability of these questionnaires have been confirmed for use in studies. The results showed that the mean score of physical performance was 60.8 (range 9.4-8) and the mean score of mental health was 62.6 (range 35.86-7). The mean scores obtained from the Quality of Life Questionnaire specific to children with cancer were 84.9 in the treatment anxiety dimension (range 0-100) and 54.2 in the procedure anxiety dimension (0-100 range). Comparing different cancer groups, it was found that 86.4% of patients with solid malignancies and 50% of blood malignancies, their cognitive dimension scores are below the seventy-fifth percentile and the physical dimension in solid malignancies below the twenty-fifth percentile. The data showed that the injury and pain scores were worse in solid malignancies, but received a better score in perception of appearance than blood malignancies. The results of this study showed that treatment methods have a significant effect on the quality of life of children with cancer, which requires the constant efforts of specialist physicians to develop new treatments with fewer side effects for these children. The researcher also states that these children should be allowed Express their concerns and fears, and pay more attention to areas of health-related quality of life that have been most affected.

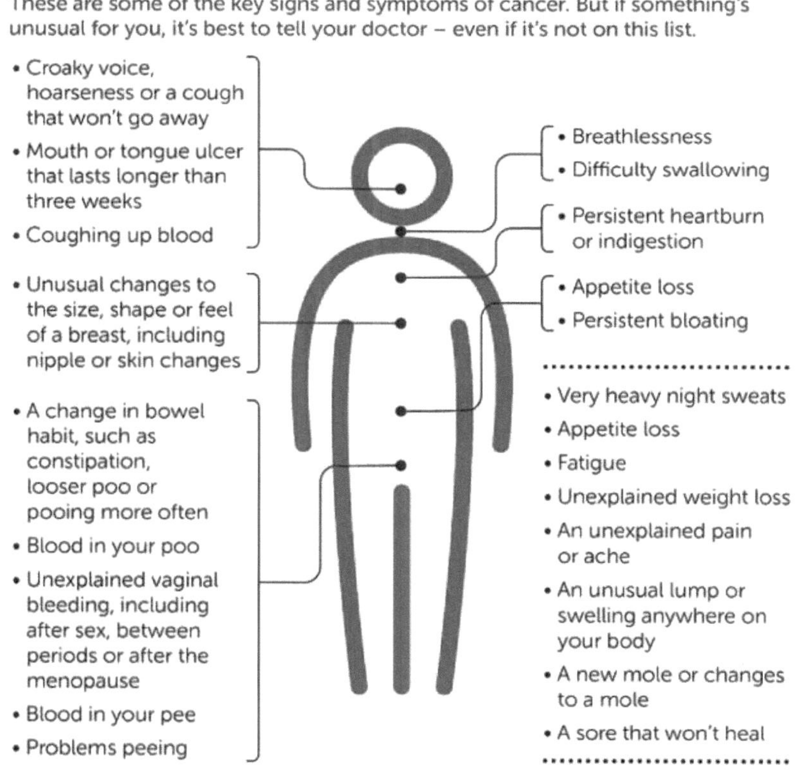

Figure 46. Signs and symptoms of cancer

Cancer in all cases affects the quality of life of patients to varying degrees. In recent years, the study of individual-social and clinical factors related to the quality of life of cancer patients has become particularly important.

In this regard, Susanto et al. (2009) conducted a cross-sectional study, with the aim of 1) comparing the quality of life of children with cancer with healthy children and 2) identifying individual social and clinical factors related to the quality of life of children with cancer in Indonesia. 77 children in the age range of 2 to 18 years who were treated participated in the study with their parents. Also, healthy children from primary and secondary schools were randomly selected and matched with the control group in terms of age and sex. Data collection tool a valid and reliable general quality of life questionnaire for children's quality of life, which consists of 4 dimensions and includes: Physical function: Factors that interfere with daily activities and exercise or cause pain or loss of energy, emotional function : Things like fear, sadness, anger, sleep or worry, educational performance: Things like attention in class, forgetfulness and absenteeism at school, social performance: Evaluates the adolescent and child's relationship with others and society.

The scoring of this questionnaire is done in 5 points by Likert method. Thus, the option always has 4 points, often 3 points, sometimes 2 points, rarely 1 point and the option never has 0 points. Then the scores are reversed and converted to 0_100 (0 = 100, 1 = 75, 2 = 50, 3 = 25, 0 = 4). Then the percentage of points obtained and the average percentage in each dimension is calculated that the higher the score, the better the quality of life. Demographic information was obtained from parents and clinical information was obtained from patients' records.

SPSS version 15 was used for data analysis. The results showed that the quality of life of children with cancer was lower than the quality of life of healthy children in all aspects (P <0.0001). Regarding the relationship between gender and quality of life in children with cancer, the findings showed that girls have a lower quality of life than boys (p <0.036). Children with lower socioeconomic status showed lower quality of life, especially in the social dimension (p <0.03). The level of education of the parents affects the quality of life of the child, children whose parents had higher education reported a higher quality of life. Also, children who had been ill for a long time reported lower quality of life in all dimensions except emotional dimension (child report: 60.08 vs. 58.2, p = 0.41, parent report: 18/8). 55 vs. 56.44, p = 0.65).

The type of cancer affects the quality of life of children. The findings of this study showed that children with leukemia showed a better quality of life, especially in the psychosocial dimension, compared to solid cancers. Older people (8 to 10 years old) had the disease and had a lower quality of life. Comparison of the results of parent-child reports in this study showed that child and parent scores were almost in the same range, although parents reported lower quality of life of the child, which can be attributed to parents' concerns about the quality of life of the child. Therefore, parents can be used as a source of information to assess the quality of life of the child and also the quality of life of children is affected by individual-social and clinical factors in different ways that these factors must be identified.

Given that leukemia is the most common cancer in children and also the type of acute lymphoblastic leukemia is the most common leukemia and its long-term survival rate has reached more than 80%, so the researchers concluded that factors related to quality of life Examine these children. In this regard, Sitarsimi et al. (2008) conducted a cross-sectional study entitled "Health-related quality of life in children with acute lymphoblastic leukemia in Indonesia. 98 children aged 2-16 years with leukemia Participated in the study with their parents, and children in critical condition were excluded from the study. For data collection, the fourth quality general quality of life questionnaires and the specific quality of life of children with cancer were used. Translated from English to Indonesia and translated back into English and then completed experimentally in 5 families by a child with leukemia and their parents, Cronbach's alpha for each instrument obtained greater than 0.70 Demographic information including: age, number of children in the family, living conditions of the child, parents 'occupation, socio-economic status, level of education of the parents was asked, and clinical information about the diagnosis, medical status was obtained from the patients' records. SPSS version 12 and to determine the relationship between Demographic and clinical variables with quality of life were paired t-test. The results of the study showed that there was no statistically significant relationship between gender, child living conditions, socio-economic status, parents' education with any of the subgroups of health-related quality of life. However, the quality of life of children aged 2-5 years was significantly lower than that of older children in the areas of diagnostic procedure anxiety, treatment anxiety and communication (P <0.05).

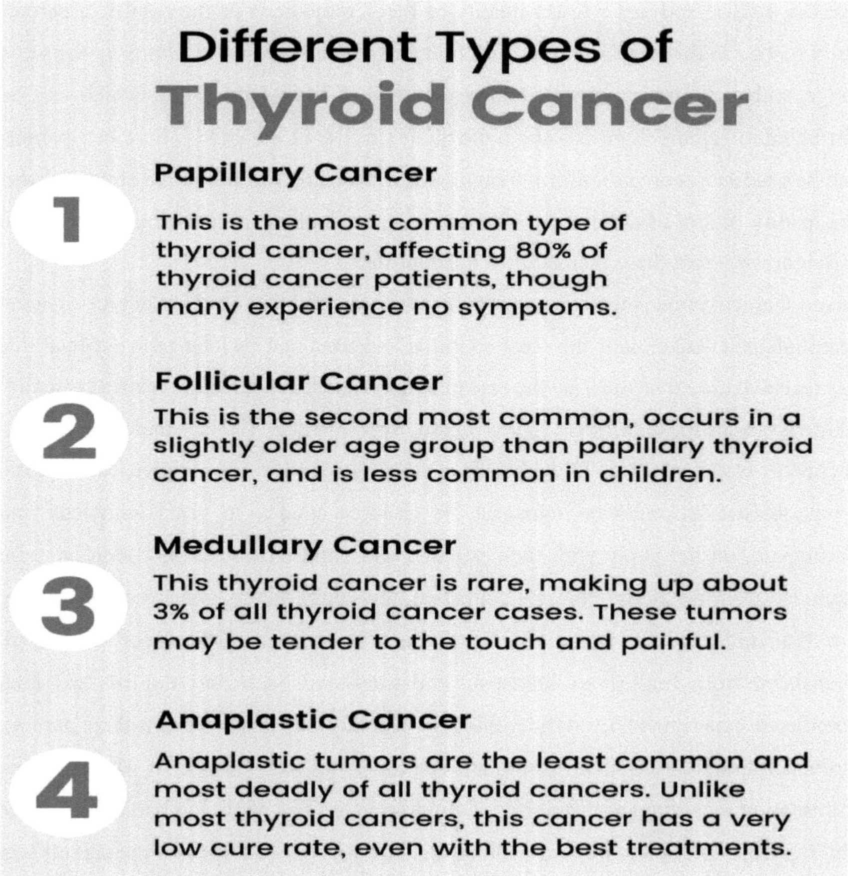

Figure 47. Thyroid Cancer: Symptoms, Diagnosis, and Treatment - Causes, symptoms, diagnosis

The total scores of both general and specific tools in the non-invasive phase of treatment were better than the invasive phase of treatment. Both tools scored better in the psychosocial dimension than in the physical dimension. There was a statistically significant relationship between children's age and decreased quality of life (P <0.05). Therefore, young children need special care to promote normal development and psychological support should be provided for the child and parents to adapt to the conditions of illness and treatment.

Recognizing quality-predicting features or conditions may help clinicians identify patients at low risk for quality of life. If these features or conditions are modifiable, implement an intervention to change them to improve quality of life. In this regard, Song et al. (2009) conducted a study with the objectives: 1) to describe the predictors of quality of life and 2) to identify children with low quality of life in Canada. Inclusion criteria were children who referred only for treatment of one type of malignancy and more than 2 months had passed since their diagnosis. To collect information, families were given a booklet containing questions about the child's quality of life and the characteristics of the child, parents and family. Child-related variables include: demographic information and parent-related variables including education level, occupation, marital status, history of chronic illness, and family-related variables: having siblings with chronic illness, family income level (more or less than $ 60,000) Per year) was. Parents were also asked to rate the severity of treatment on a 5-point scale: high severity (4 or 5) and low severity (3_1), as well as prognosis of the disease in a very good, good, and poor way. Information about the type of treatment and diagnosis was collected from the records of these patients. To evaluate the quality of life, the fourth quality children's questionnaire was used. This questionnaire has been used in previous studies and its validity and validity have been confirmed. SAS statistical program version 9 was used to analyze the data. Logistic regression was used to show the relationships between predictors and quality of life dimensions. Child sex entered the regression model due to high relationship with quality of life (p <0.0001) as well as type of cancer (p <0.0001) and family income (p <0.0001). The results of the study showed that child-related variables include: young children with leukemia diagnosis with better physical function (p <0.0001, OR = 0.37, 95% CI = 0.23_0.60) receiving chemotherapy with more severity (p <0.0008, OR = 2.34, 95% CI = 3.58-4.42) and having siblings with chronic disease (p <0.0002, OR = 2.53, 95% CI =1.54-4.15) caused poorer physical performance. A good prognosis, according to parents, and receiving less intense chemotherapy and more family income would lead to better emotional functioning. While females and having siblings with chronic disease impaired social functioning. Because the social, psychological, and physical dimensions of quality of life are affected by demographic, disease, and treatment variables, children at risk with low quality of life can be identified to provide appropriate supportive care interventions. Quality of life during treatment is affected by the toxic effects of the drug and often completely changes the daily life of the child and family. For this reason, it is recommended to evaluate the quality of life during treatment.

Having a child with cancer causes parents to spend a lot of time, energy and money on caring for the child, and as a result, they face many problems. The psychological pressures of a child's illness are such that they are unable to calm the child down and refrain from taking measures that improve the child's quality of life. If parents can adapt to the disease and its complications, they will be able to support the sick child well.

In this regard, Iser et al. (2005) conducted a study with the objectives of:

1- Determining the quality of life of mothers and children with cancer immediately after diagnosis and comparison with the control group,

2- The relationship between quality of life of mothers and child-specific concerns in the UK They gave.

Inclusion criteria include:

1- the age range of the child is 2_18 years,

2- there is only one child with cancer in the family,

3- three months have passed since the diagnosis of the disease and treatment should be done in outpatient centers.

Children with other chronic diseases as well as cognitive and neurological problems were excluded from the study. 87 children with cancer participated in the study with their mothers. In order to collect data from:

1- General Questionnaire of Children's Quality of Life, Fourth Edition, the validity and reliability of this questionnaire has been confirmed for use in studies.

2- Maternal concern tool which consists of 11 questions and examines the mother's concern about the child's future and

3- To assess the mother's health, the SF_36 quality of life tool was used, which includes examining health changes with 8 subgroups that include mental function, Examines social, mental health, vitality, pain, perception of general health, physical and social limitations. This tool is widely used in clinical research.

4- Clinical information including the type of disease and the time of its diagnosis were collected from patients' records. The questionnaires were completed by a chemotherapy nurse. SPSS version 10 was used for data analysis. The results of this study showed that compared to the healthy group, mothers of children with cancer report lower quality of life of their child and also lower quality of life than expected.

Most concerned mothers reported lower quality of life for themselves and their children in terms of physical (r = -31), emotional (r = -36) and social (r = -42) performance. There was a relationship between quality of life of children and mothers with physical (r = 0.43), emotional (r = 0.43), and social (r = 0.52) performance. The results of the study show that 3 to 5 months after the diagnosis of cancer, mothers show a lower quality of life compared to a healthy population, and mothers who were more concerned experienced a lower quality of life. The results of this study suggest that mothers can assess their child's quality of life, but this assessment also depends on their own quality of life. Mothers whose quality of life is low and who are more concerned report low quality of life of their child. These results indicate that when mothers are used to assess the quality of life of children, precautions should be taken and efforts should be made to improve the quality of life of children with cancer immediately after diagnosis by relevant organizations.

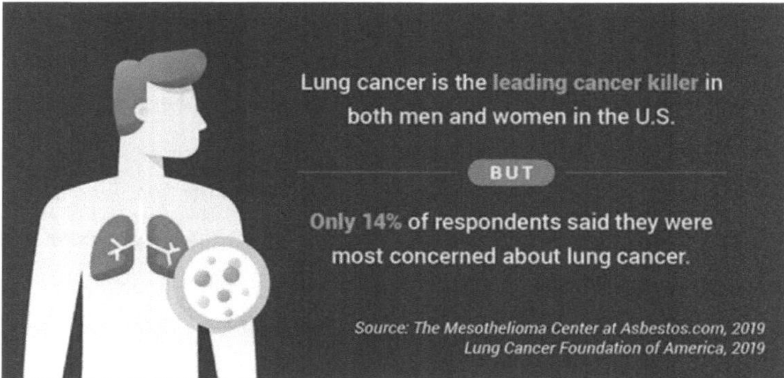

Figure 48. Deadliest Cancers Receive the Least Attention

Sayari et al., In a study entitled The Epidemiology of Pediatric Cancers in Iran, which examined cancer registry data from nine provinces, stated that the average age of children with cancer in Iran is 7.1 years. They also reported the highest age of infection in the studied provinces in the age range of 10-14 years. In another study conducted by Zol-Ali, with the aim of investigating the incidence of acute lymphoblastic cancer in children under 15 years of age in Fars's province, the average age of children diagnosed with leukemia was 7.34 years.

In the study of Stamm et al., Which was performed on 166 children with cancer with the aim of assessing the quality of life of children with cancer and the psychological reactions of parents after cancer treatment, the majority of the sample (94%) lived with their parents. The results of this study are consistent. Most mothers (49.06%) with a mean age (32.89± 6.80) years and most fathers (44.77%) with a mean age (38.58 ± 8.30) years were in the age group of 30-39 years. In this Oriental context, the average age of mothers of children with blood malignancies was reported to be 36.2 years and according to a case study, most fathers were 45 years old and most mothers were 35 years old. In this study, most mothers (33.02%) and fathers (30.84%) have high school education. In the case study, the level of education of mothers at the middle level and the level of education of fathers at the primary level, but in the study of Musk et al., Was reported at the high level.

Also, the majority of mothers (93.9%) are housewives and most fathers (35.82%) are self-employed. In Asadi's study, which aimed to investigate the effect of parent education on the quality of life of children with leukemia, most fathers (53.3%) were self-employed and the majority of mothers (97.7%) were housewives. The average monthly income in the majority of families (52.1%) was less than 300 thousand tomans. In Asadi's study, the average household income is 241,000 Tomans and in Sadghi's study, the highest household income is 182,000 Tomans. In this study, the majority of the studied units (64.32%) lived in the city.

In the study of Hashemi et al., Which was conducted to investigate the frequency distribution of different occupations of fathers in children with leukemia and non-Hodgkin's lymphoma in Yazd province, the majority of patients (63.2%) were residents of the city. In the present study, (95.78%) of the studied units had health insurance, in most of which (42.25%) had social security insurance and the majority (63.85%) were covered by Mahak Institute. Also (56.81%) families of 3_4 people, with an average (4.54 ± 1.39) had the highest percentage of samples. In Sadghi research, families of 4 people had the highest frequency.

In the study of Munir et al., In Egypt, the majority of children (34.9%) had leukemia. In the present study, the majority of the studied units (50.7%) more than one year after the diagnosis of cancer and (50.7%) more than one year after their treatment and the most common type of treatment (74.18%) chemotherapy and (48.36%) underwent chemotherapy every 21 days. In a study by Landolt et al., 96% of children were treated with chemotherapy one year after being diagnosed with cancer. The majority of children (84.51%) did not receive radiation therapy and the mean and standard deviation was the number of courses of radiation therapy (2.52 ± 7.12) that these children underwent radiation for at least 1 and at most 36 sessions.

These findings are in line with the results of the study of Stamm et al. Negative physical, cognitive, and emotional states are most affected. They also assessed the quality of life of children aged 6-14 years using the TACQOL questionnaire and found that the quality of life of children aged 6-14 years with cancer was lower in all dimensions than the quality of life of healthy children (p <0.005).

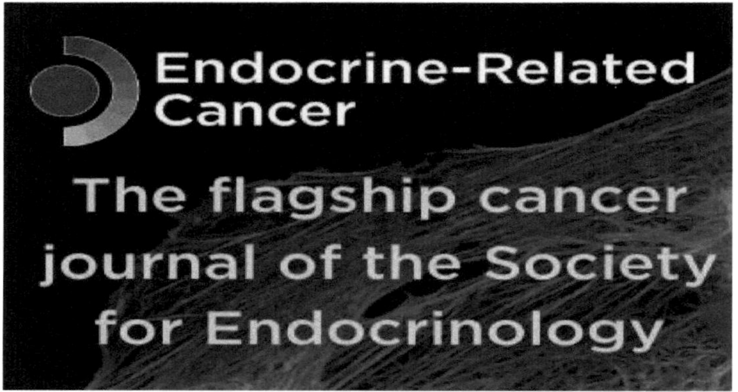

Figure 49. Endocrine-Related Cancer

In the study of Landolet et al., As in the present study, after the negative mood of children with cancer, both 6 weeks and one year after diagnosis, the lowest score of the seven dimensions of quality of life in the TNOAZL quality of life questionnaire was assigned and the total score The quality of life of the samples was reported in the low range (40). The results of Susanto et al.'s research also showed that the average quality of life scores of children with cancer in all dimensions (64.29) were lower than healthy children (80.73) (p <0.001). The results of Varney et al.'s study, which was conducted to determine the quality of life of children with chronic diseases using a general quality of life questionnaire, showed that children with chronic diseases such as cancer, asthma, diabetes, etc. compared to healthy children. They had a lower quality of life in all dimensions. Radali et al., In a study aimed at investigating the short-term and long-term effects of acute myeloblastic leukemia on the quality of life of adult patients in Italy, the cause of low quality of life in patients with acute leukemia, long-term and short-term chemotherapy treatments and treatment side effects in these patients express. It seems that physical problems due to the complications related to the disease

122

and its treatment, long course of the disease, continuous hospitalization and the need to receive frequent courses of chemotherapy cause adverse effects on the psycho-social dimensions of quality of life in these children. By developing educational plans and selecting the most appropriate treatment methods, a step can be taken to maintain and improve their quality of life.

In the study of Susanto et al., The mean and standard deviation of specific quality of life of patients with leukemia (67.0 ± 19) were reported. Also, the mean of the emotional dimension was lower than other dimensions (44.0 ± 36), which is consistent with the present study.

The results of Sang et al.'s research also showed that the average quality of life is specific (95% CI = 34.8 -94.4), in the physical dimension (54.9, 95% CI=9.4-96.9) and emotional (61.1, 95% CI=25-95) was lower than other dimensions and the average dimension of social performance (100_35 CI = 95%, 69.7) was higher than other dimensions. The results of Munier et al.'s research also showed that about one third of the samples (36.7%) reported poor quality of life. According to the researcher, psychological stress and anxiety are common consequences of cancer diagnosis and treatment that threaten the emotional dimension of these children. Also, the side effects of chemotherapy and other treatments have caused many problems in the sick child. It affects the quality of his private life.

In this regard, Stamm et al., Using a general health questionnaire (30 questions) examined the psychological response of 120 parents of children with cancer and found that parents of children with cancer experience severe psychological stress compared to the control group and health Have unfavorable generalities (p <0.001). While the results of the study by Rudenbury et al. In the United States aimed to determine the relationship between parental characteristics and quality of life of children with cancer using Beck Depression Inventory II, the symptoms of parental anxiety and stress showed that mothers have the least depressive symptoms with mean and deviation. Criteria (13.33 ± 11.57) experienced minimal symptoms of anxiety (9.04 ± 9.49) and moderate levels of stress (50.69 ± 29.95). According to the researcher, the physical and mental health of the mother and her knowledge affect how to take care of the sick child.

Therefore, when caring for children with cancer, the needs of their mothers should also be considered. Also, the difference observed with the study of Rudenbury may be due to the type of tools used.

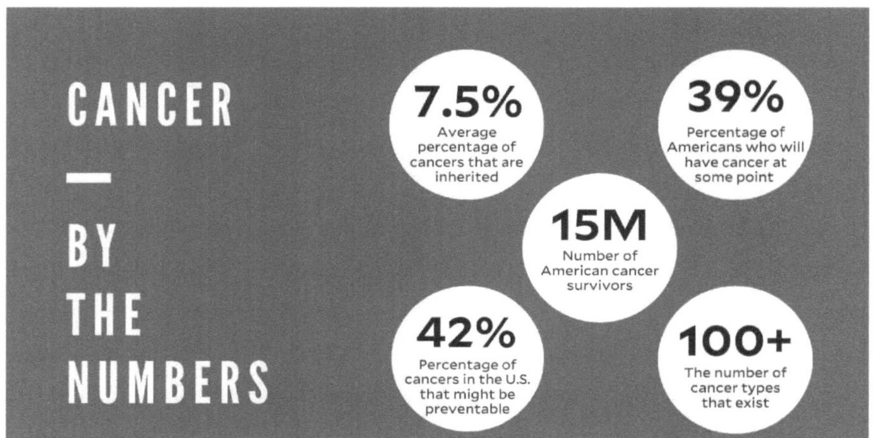

Figure 50. Cancer Causes, Symptoms, Diagnosis, Treatment, and More

The results of the findings of Vance et al., In a study aimed at determining the relationship between quality of life of children with cancer and the general health of their parents on 36 parents of children with cancer using the public health questionnaire (28 questions) showed that children with quality They had a poor life, their parents were depressed, and parents who reported a low quality of life for their children were highly stressed and considered their children more vulnerable. Iser et al. Also found that mothers who were more concerned reported lower quality of life for themselves and their children in terms of physical ($r = -31$), emotional ($r = -36$), and social ($r = -42$) functions. Another study by Yamazaki et al., Conducted on the quality of life of mothers of children with leukemia in Japan on 97 mothers of children with leukemia using the SF36 questionnaire, found that mothers whose children needed to be hospitalized regularly They have a low quality of life, especially their social functioning and mental health are endangered and they are exposed to depression.

The results of a study by Penn et al., Aimed at determining the quality of life of children with brain tumors and comparing it with healthy children in the first year after diagnosis, showed a statistically significant relationship on 37 of their mothers using Beck Depression Inventory. Between symptoms of maternal depression with quality of life related to patients' health in the physical dimension 6 months (p = 0.006, r = 0.54) and 12 months (p = 0.042, r = 0.39) after diagnosis and performance There was psychosocial (p = 0.087, r = 0.36) one month after diagnosis. It can be said that the incidence of cancer in the child and the resulting stress affect the performance of mothers and cause psychological problems in them. Therefore, families at risk of mental health problems should be identified and much attention should be paid to the issues of quality of life and psychosocial complications of treatment. P <0.0001) and specific quality of life (P <0.057).

As older children had lower health-related quality of life than younger children, so did the overall specific quality of life in younger children than in older children. In a study by Milling in Singapore, which looked at the effect of fatigue, social support, age, and adjustment patterns on the quality of life of children with cancer in 114 children using a general quality of life questionnaire, younger children who were treated for cancer were more likely than older children have a better quality of life. Susanto et al. Also stated that children aged 2-5 years with malignancy have a lower quality of specific life than children aged 10-18 years.

But the findings of Bahat et al. In a study aimed at determining the quality of life in children with brain tumors on 134 patients using a specific quality of life questionnaire, showed that younger children with brain tumors reported better specific quality of life in the psychological dimension (P<0.001). According to the researcher, older children have a better understanding of the disease process and its complications and their problem-solving power is stronger than younger children, but younger children are more vulnerable to treatment complications and have an unfavorable quality of life. As a result, more supportive measures should be considered for them.

Regarding the child sex variable, the results showed a statistically significant relationship between child sex and health-related quality of life (P <0.025) so that the average quality of life related to boys' health in cognitive dimensions (p <0.003), motor (P <0.005) and social (p <0.035) was lower than girls. In this regard, Spetcheli et al. The average quality of health-related quality of life is higher in girls than in boys.

The results of Landolt et al. Also showed that 6 weeks after the diagnosis of cancer, girls reported a better score in the independent performance dimension than boys. The results of Bahat et al.'s research also showed that girls with brain tumors received better scores in educational performance (P <0.05), while in the study of Munir et al. had life (p <0.05) so that boys gained better quality of life than girls. The results of Susanto et al. They had lower life in all dimensions (P <0.03). Perhaps this difference in results is due to the better adaptation of girls to cancer and the greater support of families for girls in the culture of our society.

Regarding the maternal education variable, the results showed a statistically significant relationship between maternal education and health-related quality of life (TAPQOL) (P <0.046). They had a low positive emotional dimension (p <0.075). In this regard, the findings of Susanto et al. Showed that there is a statistically significant relationship between parents' education level and health-related quality of life (p <0.01), so that as the level of education of parents increases, the quality of life related to the health of the child increases, but the findings of the study of Sitarsimi et al.

According to the researcher, parents are the primary caregivers in maintaining the stability and adaptation of sick children and play an important role in calming the child, preventing or exacerbating cancer complications and psychosocial complications. The quality of life of their children is of particular importance. The higher level of literacy, along with more information. Parents with higher literacy levels are more and better able to receive information such as how to care for their child, information needed for treatment, and accelerating treatment, and generally improve their child's quality of life.

Regarding the father's job variable, the results showed a statistically significant relationship between father's job and health-related quality of life (TAPQOL) (P <0.049) so that children whose fathers were unemployed and had no source of income, Poor health in social functioning (p <0.022). 300 thousand Tomans, which shows the low socio-economic status of the study units, in which Susanto et al. Showed that children with poor socio-economic status had a low quality of life, especially in the social dimension.

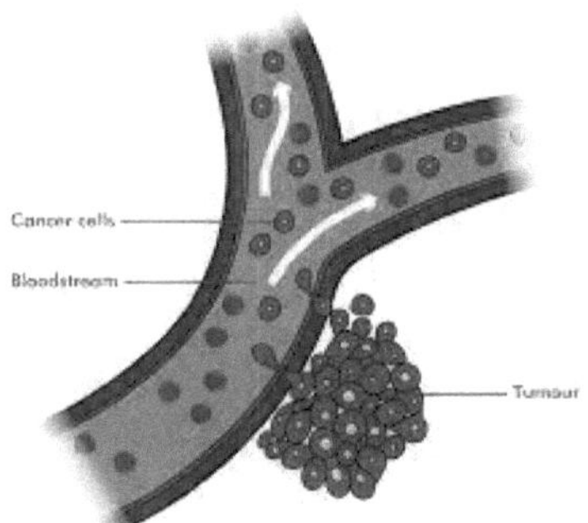

Figure 51. Secondary cancer - Macmillan Cancer Support

Another study by Zebrak et al., Entitled Psychological Consequences in Children with Leukemia and Lymphoma, showed that children with poor socioeconomic status were at higher risk for depression. The results of research by Sang et al. Also showed that children whose families have a monthly income of less than 10 They had a thousand dollars, had an unfavorable emotional performance (P <0.001). Landolt et al., However, did not report an association between socioeconomic status and quality of life.

Also, in the results of the findings of Srap et al., Who conducted a general questionnaire to identify factors related to the quality of life of adolescents cured of cancer, did not find a statistically significant relationship between father's job and quality of life of adolescents (P> 0.05). According to the child cancer researcher, it negatively affects the working situation of parents as a result of long-term care of the child, changing the role of parents and family performance.

As they may lose their jobs or work short hours, the family's source of income will be reduced. The cost of treatment, the lack of employment by parents, are very important concerns for parents of children with cancer. The support network can have a positive effect on the quality of life of children and their families through financial assistance. Regarding the variable of type of health insurance, the results showed a statistically significant relationship between the type of health insurance and health-related quality of life (TAPQOL) (P <0.022) so that children without outpatient insurance had poor quality of life related to health.

In this regard, the results of a study by Zeltzer et al., Which aimed to investigate the psychosocial consequences and health-related quality of life in childhood cancer patients, showed that environmental factors such as lack of health insurance are associated with poor quality of life. According to the researcher, the inability of the family to meet the medical needs of the child and even the basic needs of life has a direct impact on the quality of life of the child and his family. Patients and their families and the provision of services and support such as financing the treatment of these patients is essential.

Regarding the type of support system variable, the results showed a statistically significant relationship between the type of support system and the quality of private life (P <0.048), so that children supported by public aid and charities had a low quality of private life. In this regard, Milling's findings showed that there is a statistically significant relationship between social support and quality of life (P <0.001) so that children who were supported by family, friends and other institutions had a good quality of life.

According to the researcher, the assistance provided by the people and the charity association may not meet the high costs of treatment and the basic needs of these children and their families. Social institutions and designing programs to help such families, counseling and professional help to solve the problems of these families is essential. Therefore, by improving the quality of life of family members and providing better support to patients, the quality of life of patients also increases.

Regarding the cancer variable, the results showed a statistically significant relationship between the type of cancer and health-related quality of life (P <0.0001), so that children with Wilms' tumor and brain tumor were related to quality of life compared to other types of cancer. They had poor health in social dimensions (P <0.000), physical (P <0.000), negative emotional (P <0.026) and positive emotional (P <0.007).

In this regard, the results of a study by Musk et al., Entitled Health-Related Quality of Life Factors in Childhood Cancer Healers, which was performed on 86 children aged 2-18 years, using the General Quality of Life Questionnaire, showed a risk. Most children with brain tumors threaten the health-related quality of life in the psychosocial dimension.

Also, the results of the findings of Begoul et al. They reported in social, emotional, physical and educational dimensions (p <0.001). Warren et al. In the study of Song et al., Children with leukemia (71.29±18.1) had a better quality of life than other types of cancer, especially in terms of physical function (66.21±19.22). According to the researcher, each of the cancers causes certain complications and problems that may be different from other cancers. Therefore, it can be said that the quality of life in children with cancer is different from different types of cancer, and these differences can help to identify more vulnerable children and their needs and intervention to improve the quality of life.

Regarding the type of treatment variable, the results showed a statistically significant relationship between the type of treatment and health-related quality of life (P <0.015). P <0.009), social (p <0.047) and motor (p <0.032). In this regard, the findings of Bahat et al. Showed that patients undergoing combination therapies such as radiation therapy and chemotherapy They had a lower quality of life than those who received radiation therapy alone (65) and Munir et al. Found that the type of treatment was significantly related to quality of life (p <0.05). They underwent surgery and had a better quality of life than children who received chemotherapy and radiation. They harm the child's life, so take steps to achieve better treatments or treatments. Supportive is useful to reduce side effects.

Regarding the duration of treatment, the results showed a statistically significant relationship between the duration of treatment and quality of life related to health (P <0.0001), so that children who are treated for less than a year, in physical dimensions (P <0.039) (P <0.000), motor (p <0.000), social (p <0.005) and positive emotional (p

<0.0001) are most affected. In this regard, the results of research by Varney et al. Showed that children who had just been diagnosed with cancer and had been treated for a short time reported a lower quality of life than children who had been treated for a long time.

Preventable cancers

More than 40 percent of cancer cases can be prevented, the American Cancer Society finds in a new report. Here is a list of things people can change and their share of cancer cases:

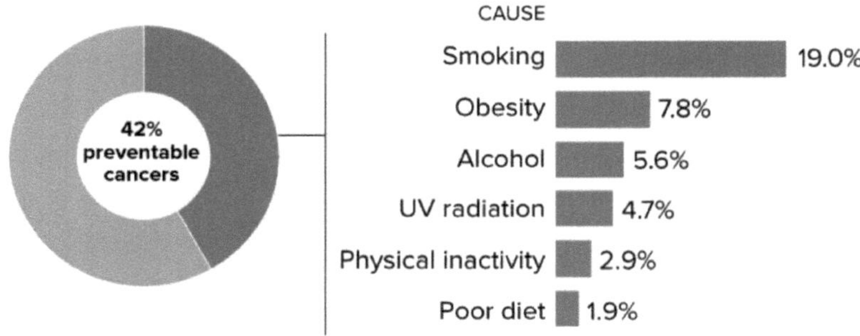

Figure 52. Fresh look at cancer shows smoking, obesity top causes

However, the results of Musk et al.'s study, which was performed to assess the quality of life of children with brain tumors and leukemia using the General Cancer Quality of Life Questionnaire, showed a statistically significant relationship between the duration of treatment and quality of life (P <0.03). Children with brain tumors who were treated for less than a year had a better quality of life than children who were treated for more than a year (P <0.001), while children with leukemia with a Years or more after treatment, they had a better quality of life. The results may be due to the aggressiveness of the anticancer treatment in the first year of treatment.

Regarding the variable duration of the disease, the results showed a statistically significant relationship between the duration of the disease and health-related quality of life (P <0.0001) so that children who are less than one year of their disease duration Passage in physical dimensions (p <0.007), motor (p <0.000), social (p <0.001), negative emotional (p <0.038) and positive emotional (p <0.0001) quality Health-related lives are more harmed. Contrary to the results of the present study, Rudenbury et al. Showed that there is no statistically significant relationship between the duration of the disease and the quality of life of the child (p <0.63, r = 0.12). It can be said that by diagnosing the disease and starting treatment, the stressors caused by the disease and its treatment cause more negative consequences on physical and mental health and cause patients to experience less happiness and adaptability. Therefore, they are expected to have a lower quality of life compared to patients who have been diagnosed for a longer period of time.

Regarding the interval between chemotherapy courses, the results showed a statistically significant relationship between the distance between chemotherapy courses and health-related quality of life (P <0.0001) and specific quality of life (P <0.056). So that children who received chemotherapy every day, in physical dimensions (p <0.0001), motor (p <0.0001), social (p <0.015), negative emotional (P <0.003) and positive (p <0.0001) had low quality of life related to health and also these children had low specific quality of life in emotional (p <0.0001) and social (p <0.039) dimensions. In this regard, the results of the findings of Yaris et al. Showed that the intensity of treatment has a significant effect on the quality of life of children with cancer, so that children who were frequently treated with chemotherapy had a lower quality of life (P <0.007). In addition to cancer cells, chemotherapy drugs also damage healthy cells and cause side effects, so the more consecutive courses of treatment, the greater the damage to health and quality of life.

Regarding the variable number of radiation therapy courses, the results showed a statistically significant relationship between the number of radiation therapy courses and health-related quality of life (P <0.007) and specific quality of life (P <0.016), so that children who More courses were undergoing radiation therapy. In the physical dimension (p <0.025), the quality of life was related to health, and in the dimension of treatment complications (p <0.0001) and the psychological dimension (p <0.040), the specific quality of life was more damaged. In this regard, the results of the research of Bahat et al. Showed that children who received radiation therapy but did not receive chemotherapy had a lower general quality of life in all aspects than other treatments (P <0.05) and also They had a lower specific quality of life in the psychological dimension (P <0.05). It can be said that radiation therapy also affects healthy cells and has side effects, so it can affect the physical dimension of quality of life.

On the other hand, if several treatments are used to treat cancer, it is a sign that it is high risk, so the psychological dimension. It also affects the quality of life. Regression analysis showed a statistically significant relationship between the age of the child and the quality of life related to health (p <0.001), so that with increasing one year of age, the average quality of life is related. With health it decreases by 1.18.

There was also a statistically significant relationship between age and mean quality of private life (p <0.046), so that with increasing the age of the child by 5 years, the probability of quality of private life becomes more favorable by 1.59. In this regard, the study of Sang Et al. Showed that older children had better health-related quality of life (p <0.003).

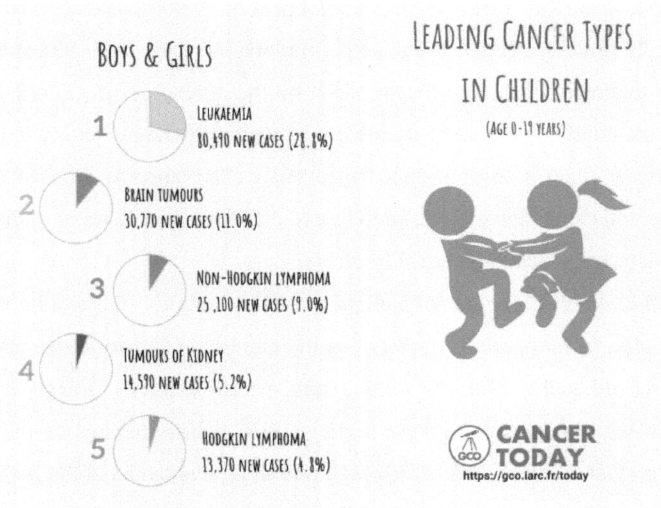

Figure 53. Global Cancer Observatory

In Varney et al.'s study, older children also had healthier health-related quality of life. The results of Munier et al.'s findings also showed that age is highly correlated with quality of private life (p <0.05). Older children reported a better quality of private life than younger children.

Sitarsimi et al. also showed that younger children had a more unfavorable quality of life in psychological and social dimensions (p <0.05). According to the researcher, these results may be due to the adaptation of older children to the complications of cancer and treatment than younger children, which makes older children have a better quality of life. Therefore, younger children need special care when performing therapeutic interventions. In contrast, older children experience health-related quality of life due to greater social development and interactions, feelings of lack of self-confidence, and frequent absences from school due to illness, frequent hospitalizations, and the realization that they will never be without symptoms.

Regression analysis showed a statistically significant relationship between maternal general health and quality of private life (P <0.047), so that in exchange for a decrease in maternal general health, the desired quality of private life decreases by 1.06.

In this regard, the findings of Landolt et al., Which were conducted to assess the psychological adjustment of parents using a brief symptom questionnaire on parents of children with cancer, found that children whose parents had better mental adjustment, their children showed less cognitive problems. (p <0.05). Also, in the acute phase of treatment, parental psychological stress had a negative effect on the emotional dimension of the child, but no statistically significant relationship was found. In another study by Stamm et al. To evaluate psychosocial indicators of health-related quality of life in children with cancer in 2 months after treatment on 150 parents of children with cancer using a general health questionnaire (30 questions Showed that parents who were more stressed reported more problems in their child's physical function (p <0.001). Also, the results of the findings of Begoul et al. (P <0.001), social (P <0.001) and educational (P <0.001) found a statistically significant relationship so that children whose parents had good mental health had a good quality of life. According to the researcher, the presence of a child with a chronic disease such as cancer in the family is a threatening factor that can affect the mental health of parents, especially mothers. Psychiatry should be established for screening and early treatment of mothers, in order to improve the quality of life of their sick children by treating depression and improving mothers' performance.

Regression analysis showed a statistically significant relationship between the duration of the disease and quality of life related to health (p <0.045), so that children less than one year after the onset of the disease, 2.42 The chances of a good quality of life in them are reduced. This finding is in line with the results of a study by Landolt et al. In this study, the quality of life of the samples was measured by a quality-of-life questionnaire 6 weeks and one year after diagnosis. The results of this study showed that the quality-of-life score of children with leukemia decreased in 6 weeks and one year after diagnosis in motor, physical and emotional dimensions and this decrease in 6 weeks after diagnosis was more severe than the end of the first year.

The results of the study by Susanto et al. also showed that children who were ill for a longer period of time reported better emotional functioning. However, in the study of Munir et al., No significant difference was found between the duration of the disease and the quality of specific life (p <0.16).

According to the researcher, these findings indicate that the psychological problems caused by the diagnosis of the disease in the early stages of diagnosis and the shock created in the sick child due to aggressive treatment methods and complications of the disease and treatment can be quality of life related to the health of the sick child. Make undesirable. On the other hand, with the passage of time and the increase in the duration of the disease, the patient's acceptance of the disease increases and he comes to terms with his problems and finds appropriate solutions, thus not having the anxiety and anxiety of the early disease.

Regression analysis showed a significant relationship between the mean health-related quality of life and the interval between courses of chemotherapy (p <0.006), so that children who receive chemotherapy every day compared to those who every 21 Once a day undergoing chemotherapy, the quality of public life becomes 7.9 times worse. Also, there was a statistically significant relationship between the distance between chemotherapy courses and the mean quality of specific life (p <0.035) so that children who receive chemotherapy every day compared to those who received chemotherapy every 21 days by 2.81 the quality of private life becomes more unfavorable.

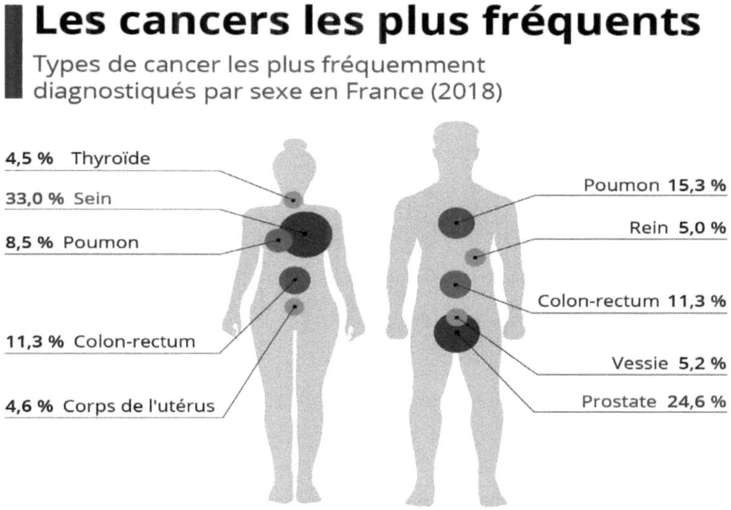

Les cancers les plus fréquents

Types de cancer les plus fréquemment diagnostiqués par sexe en France (2018)

Figure 54. What are the most diagnosed forms of cancer in France?

In this regard, the results of research by Sang Et al. Showed that children undergoing severe chemotherapy treatment have a quality of life associated with poor health, especially in the dimensions of physical and motor function (p = 0.0008, 95% CI=1.42-3.85, OR =2.34).

In the study of Landolet et al., Children who were severely treated with chemotherapy in the dimensions of physical function (r = -0.3, p <0.05), motor (p = 0.01, r = -0.34) and Positively emotional (p = 0.032 - (r = most injured). The study of Sitarsimi et al. Emotional (61±21) and education (47 ± 26) quality of life related to health as well as in the dimensions of treatment (59 ± 31), psychological (34 ± 34) and social (43 ± 34) specific quality of life were more damaged.

The results show that severe and invasive treatments such as chemotherapy with the unwanted problems it causes, reduce the quality of life of the sick child and make appropriate interventions to reduce the side effects of chemotherapy. Regression analysis showed a statistically significant relationship between the number of radiotherapy courses and quality of life related to health, so that children who received radiation therapy between 1-19 sessions, on average, those who did not receive radiation therapy, 5.31 The chances of a health-related quality of life are reduced by 5 times.

Also, a statistically significant relationship was observed between the number of courses of radiation therapy and the mean quality of specific life (p <0.035), so that children who received radiation therapy between 1-19 sessions, compared to those who did not receive radiation therapy by 2.95 The chances of a good quality of life are reduced. Also, children who received equal or more than 20 sessions of radiation therapy had a 9.07 times more poor quality of private life than those who did not receive radiation therapy.

In this regard, the results of Begol et al. Showed that children who received radiation therapy had poorer educational performance than children who did not receive radiation (p <0.001).

Another study by Spatley et al., Entitled Quality of Life in Children and Adolescents Cured of Cancer in London, using the Child Health Questionnaire, found that patients treated with radiation therapy outperformed other quality-of-life treatments. They had lower (p <0.005) and their physical and mental-social dimensions were more damaged. According to the researcher, the results of the mentioned studies indicate this: Children who receive radiation therapy are more prone to harm, which increases with the number of radiation therapy sessions. As a result, the development of strategies for continuous follow-up in groups Special from patients is essential.

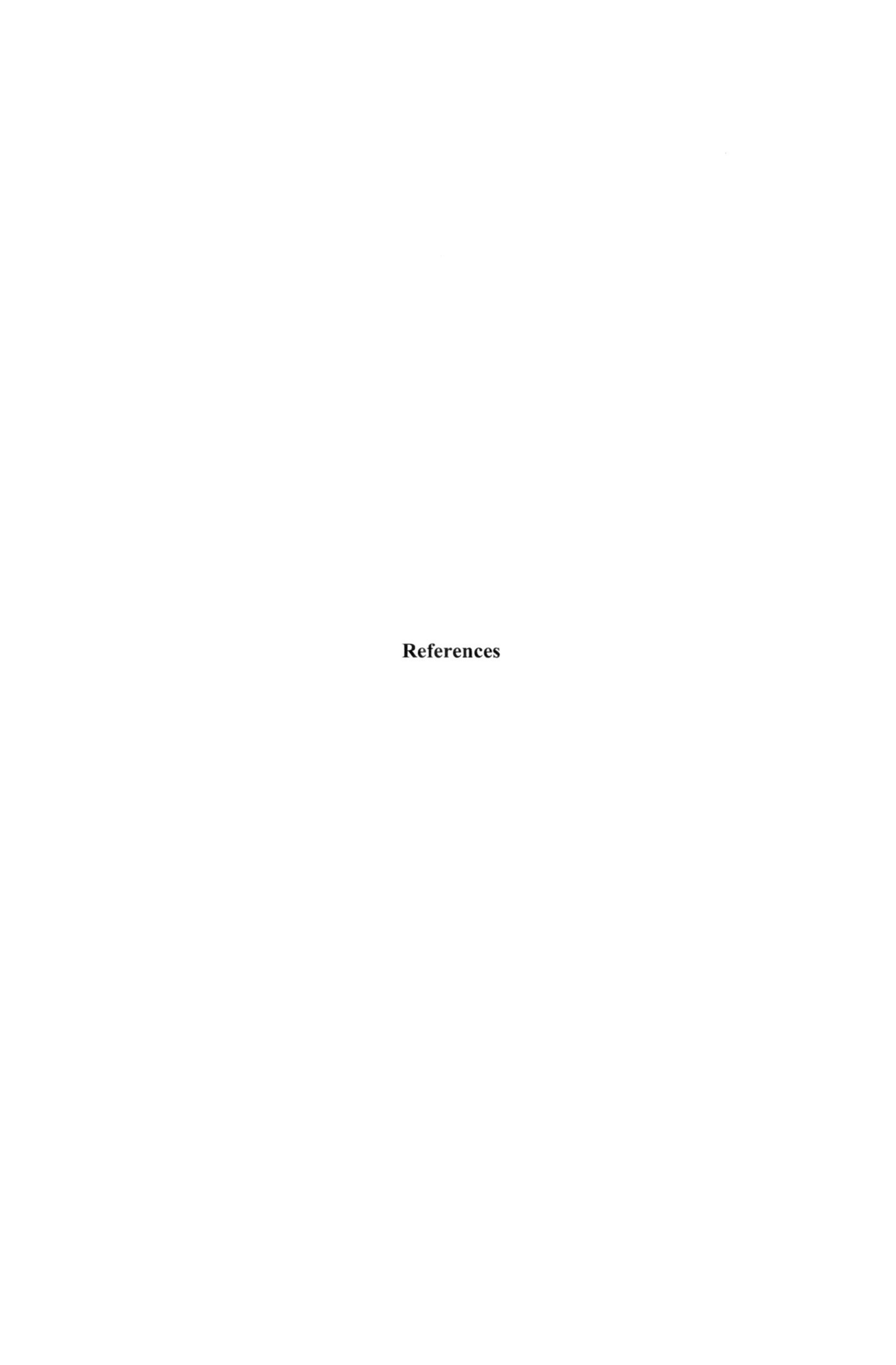

References

A. Arroliga, R. Matthay. The role of bronchoscopy in lung cancer. Clin. Chest Med., 1993, 14, 87-98.

A. J. Alberg, M. V. Brock, J. M. Samet. Epidemiology of lung cancer: looking to the future. J. Clin. Oncol., 2005, 23, 3175-3185.

Aguilar-Ruiz JS, Riquelme JC, Toro M. Evolutionary Learning of Hierarchical Decision Rules, in IEEE Transactions on Systems 2003; 33(2): 324-34.

Andres C, Pena R, Sipper M. Designing Breast Cancer Diagnostic Systems via aHybrid Fuzzy-Genetic Methodology, IEEE International Fuzzy Systems Conference 1999; 1: 135-9.

Ashlaghi A, Pour Ebrahimi A, Ebrahimi M, Ahmad L. Using data mining techniques for prediction breast cancer recurrence, Iranian Journal of Breast Disease 2013; 5(4): 23-34.

Bewick M, Krause A. Her-2 Expression is a prognostic factor in patient with metastatic breast cancer treated with combination of High-dose cyclophosphamide, paclitaxel, Mitoxatrone and autologus Blood stem cell support. Bone Marrow transplantation 2001 Apr; 27(8): 847-53.

Bland KI, Verzerides MP, Copeland III EM. Breast In: Schwartz SI, Shires GT, Spencer FC, editors. Principles of surgery. 7 th ed. New York: McGraw Hill; 1999. P. 554-92.

Brodwicz I, Kandior O, Anti Her-2/Neu Antibody induces Apoptosis in Her-2/Neu overexpressing breast cancer cells independently from P53 status. British journal of cancer 2001 Nov; 85(11): 1764-70

C. E. Kim, K. M. Tchou-Wong, W. N. Rom. Sputum-Based Molecular Biomarkers for the Early Detection of Lung Cancer: Limitations and Promise. Cancers, 2011, 3, 2975-2989.

Carr JA, Havstad S. The association of Her2 amplification with breast cancer recurrence. Archieves of surgery 2000 Des; 135(12): 1469- 74.

Cho HS, Mason K, Ramyor KK, Stanly AM, Gabell SB. Structure of the Extracellular region of Her-2 alone and in complex with herceptin Fab. Nature 2003 Feb 13; 421(6924): 756-60.

Colon E, Rayer JS, Gonzalez Keelan C, Climent peris C. Prevalence of steroied Receptor and Her-2/Neu in Breast biopsies of women living in puertorico. Puertorice health-sciences Journal 2002; 21(4): 299-303.

D. Hayes, H. Secrist, C. Bangur, T. Wang, X. Zhang, D. Harlan, G. Goodman, R. Houghton, D. Persing, B. Zehentner. Multigene real-time PCR detection of circulating tumor cells in peripheral blood of lung cancer patients. Anticancer Res., 2006, 26, 1567-1576.

Daly JM, Bertagnolli M, Decosse JJ, Morton DM. Oncology in: Schwartz SI, Shires GT, Spencer FC, editors. Principles of surgery, 7th ed. New York: MC-Graw Hill; 1999. P. 308-9, 323.

Endo A, Shibata T, Tanaka H. Comparison of seven algorithms to predict breast cancer survival, Biomedical Soft Computing and Human Sciences 2008; 13(2): 6-11.

F. Liu, P. Xiao, H. Fang, H. Dai, L. Qiao, Y. Zhang. Single-walled carbon nanotube-based biosensors for the detection of volatile organic compounds of lung cancer. Physica E, 2011, 44, 367-372.

F. R. Hirsch, W. A. Franklin, A. F. Gazdar, P. A. Bunn. Early detection of lung cancer: clinical perspectives of recent advances in biology and radiology. Clin. Cancer Res., 2001, 7, 5-22.

F. Taher, N. Werghi, H. Al-Ahmad, C. Donner. Extraction and Segmentation of Sputum Cells for Lung Cancer Early Diagnosis. J. Algorithms, 2013, 6, 512-531.

G. Ellison, G. Zhu, A. Moulis, S. Dearden, G. Speake, R. M. Cormack. EGFR mutation testing in lung cancer: a review of available methods and their use for analysis of tumour tissue and cytology samples. J. Clin. Pathol., 2013, 66, 79-89.

G. Peng, M. Hakim, Y. Y. Broza, S. Billan, R. Abdah-Bortnyak, A. Kuten, U. Tisch, H. Haick. Detection of lung, breast, colorectal, and prostate cancers from exhaled breath using a single array of nanosensors. Brit. J. Cancer, 2010, 103, 542-551.

G. Peng, U. Tisch, O. Adams, M. Hakim, N. Shehada, Y. Y. Broza, S. Billan, R. Abdah-Bortnyak, A. Kuten, H. Haick. Diagnosing lung cancer in exhaled breath using gold nanoparticles. Nat. nanotechnol., 2009, 4, 669-673.

G. S. Wright, M. E. Gruidl. Early detection and prevention of lung cancer. Curr. Opin. Oncol., 2000, 12, 143-148.

Ganji MF, Abadeh MS. Parallel Fuzzy Rule Learning Using an ACO-Based Algorithm for Medical Data Mining, IEEE Fifth. International conference on Bio InnspiredCompting: theories and Applications 2010; 573-81.

Gerber B, Krause A. Effectiveness of herceptin in patient with locally recurrence breast cancer after cardiac failure caused by sever cytotoxic pretreatment. Oncology 2001; 61(4): 271-4.

H. Zhang, D. Yee, C. Wang. Quantum dots for cancer diagnosis and therapy: biological and clinical perspectives. Nanomedicine-UK, 2008, 3, 83-91.

Herdy V. Education: a key factor in fighting breast cancer. New York: Inter press services 1998; 1.

Huge OF, Yamauch H. Circulating Her-2 extracellular domain as a prognostic factor with metastatic breast cancer. Clinical cancer research 2001 Sep; 7(9): 2605-7.

Iglehort JD, Kaelin CM. Breast. In: Tounsend courtney MJR, Beauchamp R.D, Mark Evers B. SABISTON text book of surgery. Philadelphia, pennesylvania: W.B. Saunders company; 2001. P. 568-90.

Iran Ministry of Health & Medical Education. Diseases management center, cancer office. Country report of cancer cases. Tehran: KelkZarrin Press 2004; 16. Sadeghnezhad F, NiknamiSh, Ghaffari M, Effect of health education methods on promoting breast self-examination (BSE), Journal of Birjand University of Medical Sciences 2009; 15(4): 38-48.

Iran Ministry of Health & Medical Education. Health deputy, Family Health office, adult health and women office. Primary report of breast cancer screening 1st ed. Tehran: Ministry of Health & Medical Education 2000; 18-36.

J. D. Minna, J. A. Roth, A. F. Gazdar. Focus on lung cancer. Cancer cell, 2002, 1, 49-52.

J. Drbohlavova, V. Adam, R. Kizek, J. Hubalek. Quantum dots—characterization, preparation and usage in biological systems. Int. j. mol. sci., 2009, 10, 656-673.

Jain R, Abraham A. A Comparative Study of Fuzzy Classification Methods on Breast Cancer Data, Australas Phys Eng Sci Med 2004; 27(4): 213-8.

Jain R, Mazumdar J. A Genetic Algorithm based Nearest Neighbor Classification to Breast Cancer Diagnosis, Australasian Physical & Engineering Sciences in Medicine 2003; 26(1):6-11.

Joen Sun H, Isola J, Lundin M, Salminen T, Holli K, Kataja V. Amplification of erb-b2 and erb-b2 expression are superior to ER status as risk factor for distance recurrence in patient T1N0M0 breast cancer. Clinical cancer research 2003 M0; 9(3): 223-309.

John GH, Langley P. Estimating continuous distributions in bayesian classifiers. In Proceedings of the Eleventh Conference on Unccertanity in Artificial Intelligence 1995; 338-345.

Keramatee K, Ghorbanian M, Abbasnia V, PazirehN, Alipour H, Effect of Flunixin as a Cox Inhibitor on Prevention and Cure of Breast Cancer in Female Wistar Rat, the Horizon of Medical Sciences 2010; 15 (4): 24-32.

Kim YS, Kanopler SN. Her-2 Overexpresion as a poor prognostic factor for patient with metastatic breast cancer undergoing high-dose chemotherapy with Autologus stemcell transplantation. Clinical cancer research. 2001 Dec; 7(12): 4003-12.

Kotsiantis SB. Supervised machin leaming: a reviw of classification techniques, informatica 31, 2007; 249-68.

L. Zhang, D. Lv, W. Su, Y. Liu, Y. Chen, R. Xiang. Detection of cancer biomarker with nanotechnology. Am. J. Biochem. Biotechnol., 2013, 9, 71-89.

M. Hu, J. Yan, Y. He, H. Lu, L. Weng, S. Song, C. Fan, L. Wang. Ultrasensitive, multiplexed detection of cancer biomarkers directly in serum by using a quantum dot-based microfluidic protein chip. ACS Nano, 2009, 4, 488-494.

Moller P, Wallin H, Knudesen LE. Oxidative stress associated psychological stress and life-style factor. Chem Bio Interact 1996; 102: 1-36.

Mousavi SM, Montazeri A, Mohagheghi MA, MousaviJarrahi A, Harirchi I, Najafi M, Ebrahimi M. Breast cancer in Iran: an epidemiological review. Breast J 2007; 13: 383-91.

N. S. Ramgir, A. Zajac, P. K. Sekhar, L. Lee, T. A. Zhukov, S. Bhansali. Voltammetric detection of cancer biomarkers exemplified by interleukin-10 and osteopontin with silica nanowires. J. Phys. Chem. C, 2007, 111, 13981-13987.

N. Sinha, J. T. Yeow. Carbon nanotubes for biomedical applications. IEEE T. NanoBiosci., 2005, 4, 180-195.

Namiki M. Antioxidant /antimutagenes in foods. Crit Rev. food SciNutr 1990; 29: 273-300.

Nguyen AN, Lawley MJ, Hansen DP, Bowman RV, Clarke BE, Duhig EE, Colquist S. Symbolic rule-based classification of lung cancer stages from free-text pathology reports. J Am Med Inform Assoc 2010; 17(4):440-5.

P. K. Sekhar, N. S. Ramgir, R. K. Joshi, S. Bhansali. Selective growth of silica nanowires using an Au catalyst for optical recognition of interleukin-10. Nanotechnology, 2008, 19, 5502-5508.

Parkin DM, Bray F, Ferlay J, Pisani P. Global cancer statistics 2002. CA Cancer J Clin 2005; 55(2): 74-108.

R. Hubaux, D. D. Becker-Santos, K. S. Enfield, S. Lam, W. L. Lam, V. D. Martinez. Arsenic, asbestos and radon: emerging players in lung tumorigenesis. J. Environ. Health, 2012, 11, 89-100.

R. M. Reilly. Carbon nanotubes: potential benefits and risks of nanotechnology in nuclear medicine. J. Nucl. Med., 2007, 48, 1039-1042.

Rosai J. Surgical pathology, Elsevier Inc. 9th edition Piladerphia 2004; 380-92.

S. Nie, Y. Xing, G. J. Kim, J. W. Simons. Nanotechnology applications in cancer. Annu. Rev. Biomed. Eng., 2007, 9, 257-288.

S. r. Ji, C. Liu, B. Zhang, F. Yang, J. Xu, J. Long, C. Jin, D. l. Fu, Q. x. Ni, X. j. Yu. Carbon nanotubes in cancer diagnosis and therapy. BBA-Rev. Cancer, 2010, 1806, 29-35.

S. Y. Luo, D. C. Lam. Oncogenic driver mutations in lung cancer. Transl. Respir. Med., 2013, 1, 6-13.

T. K. Sethi, M. N. El-Ghamry, G. H. Kloecker. Radon and lung cancer. Clin. Adv. Hematol. Oncol., 2012, 10, 157-164.

T. Ozlu, Y. Bubul. Smoking and lung cancer. Tüberküloz ve Toraks Dergisi, 2005, 53, 200-209.

W. Yang, P. Thordarson, J. J. Gooding, S. P. Ringer, F. Braet. Carbon nanotubes for biological and biomedical applications. Nanotechnology, 2007, 18, 412-420.

Wang Rodrigez J, Cross K, Callagher S, Ojahanbin M, Armstrong JM. Male breast cancer correlation of ER, PR, Her-2 and P53 with treatment and survival a study of 65 cases. Modern pathology 2002 Aug; 15(8): 853-61. 7- Lipton A, Ali SM, Leitzel K. Eleuated serum Her-2 level predicts decrease response to hormone thrapy in metatatic breast cancer. Journal of clinical oncology 2002 Mar; 20(6): 1467- 72.

Wilson CM, Tobin S, Young RC. The exploding worldwide cancer burden: the impact of cancer on women. Int J Gynecol Cancer 2004; 14: 1-11.

Wilton CJ, Reeve JR, Going JJ, Cooke TG, Bortlett JM. Expression of the Her1-4 Family of receptor tyrosine kinase in breast cancer. Journal of pathology 2003; 200(3): 290-7.

Wuy Kan H, Chilar R. Prognostic value of plasma Her-2/Neu in African American and Hispanic woman with breast cancer. International journal of oncology 1999 Jun; 14(6): 1021-37. 13- Hehl EM. Opinion on the use of Anti-tumor druge trastuzumab (Herception) in patient with metastatic breast cancer. International journal of clinical pharmacology and thrapeutics. 2001 Nov; 39(4): 503-6.

Y. E. Choi, J.W. Kwak, J. W. Park. Nanotechnology for early cancer detection. Sensors, 2010, 10, 428-455.

Z. L. Wang, R. P. Gao, Z. W. Pan, Z. R. Dai. Nano-scale mechanics of nanotubes, nanowires, and nanobelts. Adv. Eng. Mater., 2001, 3, 657-661.

Zhou Zh, Jiang Y. Medical diagnosis with C4.5 Rule preceded by artificial neural network ensemble. IEEE Trans InfTechnol Biomed 2003; 7(1): 37-42.

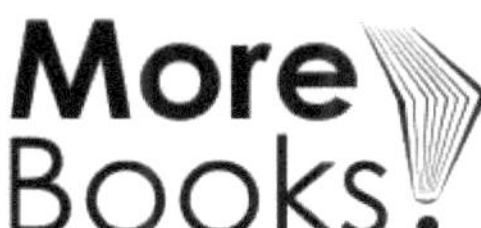

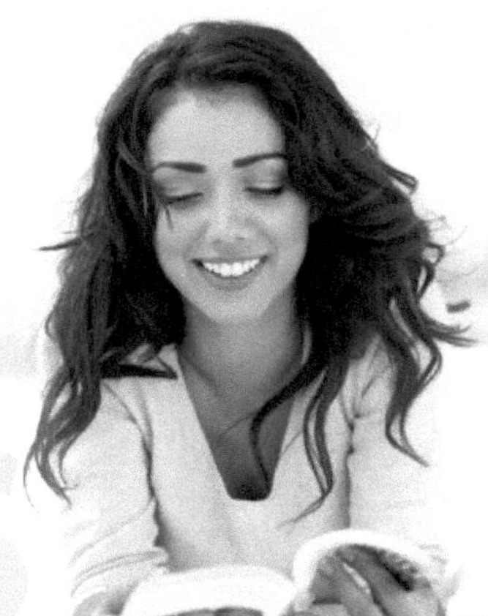

I **want** morebooks!

Buy your books fast and straightforward online - at one of world's fastest growing online book stores! Environmentally sound due to Print-on-Demand technologies.

Buy your books online at
www.morebooks.shop

Kaufen Sie Ihre Bücher schnell und unkompliziert online – auf einer der am schnellsten wachsenden Buchhandelsplattformen weltweit! Dank Print-On-Demand umwelt- und ressourcenschonend produzi ert.

Bücher schneller online kaufen
www.morebooks.shop

KS OmniScriptum Publishing
Brivibas gatve 197
LV-1039 Riga, Latvia
Telefax: +371 686 204 55

info@omniscriptum.com
www.omniscriptum.com

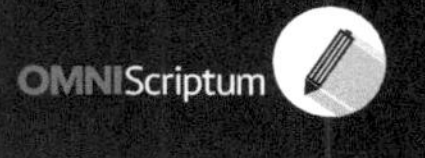

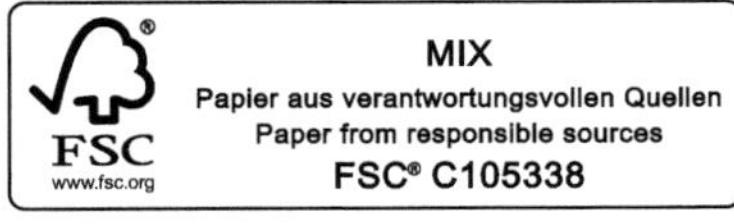

Printed by Books on Demand GmbH, Norderstedt / Germany